SKIN GRAFTING

John W. Skouge, M.D.

Director
Division of Dermatologic Surgery
Departments of Dermatology and Otolaryngology/
Head and Neck Surgery
The Johns Hopkins Medical Institutions
Baltimore, Maryland

Illustrated by Mary A. Jordan, M.A.

CHURCHILL LIVINGSTONE
New York, Edinburgh, London, Melbourne

Library of Congress Cataloging-in-Publication Data

Skouge, John W.
    Skin Grafting / John W. Skouge ; illustrated by Mary A. Jordan.
       p.   cm. — (Practical manuals in dermatologic surgery)
    Includes bibliographical references.
    Includes index.
    ISBN 0-443-08706-7
    1. Skin-grafting.   2. Surgery, Outpatient.   I. Title.
  II. Series.
    [DNLM: 1. Ambulatory Care. 2. Skin Transplantation—methods.   WO
  610 S628s]
  RD121.S58 1991
  617.4′ 770592—dc20
  DNLM/DLC
  for Library of Congress   90-2421
                                      CIP

© **Churchill Livingstone Inc. 1991**

Distributed in the United Kingdom by Churchill Livingstone, Robert Stevenson House, 1–3 Baxter's Place, Leith Walk, Edinburgh EH1 3AF, and by associated companies, branches, and representatives throughout the world.

Accurate indications, adverse reactions, and dosage schedules for drugs are provided in this book, but it is possible that they may change. The reader is urged to review the package information data of the manufacturers of the medications mentioned.

The Publishers have made every effort to trace the copyright holders for borrowed material. If they have inadvertently overlooked any, they will be pleased to make the necessary arrangements at the first opportunity.

Acquisitions Editor: *Beth Kaufman Barry*
Copy Editor: *Marian Ryan*
Production Designer: *Marci Jordan*
Production Supervisor: *Sharon Tuder*

Printed in the United States of America

First published in 1991

FOREWORD

As surgery becomes a more integral part of the practice of dermatology, it is necessary that the literature and training keep pace. Although surgical skills are currently being taught on a regular basis as part of the residency core curriculum, few "how to" manuals exist. Additionally, many practicing dermatologists wish to increase their surgical knowledge. The courses are available, but detailed instructional manuals for day to day office use are lacking.

In this spirit, this series, *Practical Manuals in Dermatologic Surgery*, was conceived. The manuals are designed to be "user friendly." Historical aspects and basic science information are excluded or mentioned only as absolutely necessary. The focus is purely on telling the reader how to perform specific procedures in a logical stepwise fashion.

Dermatologic surgery covers a wide gamut of areas; not all dermatologists wish to pursue every facet. Therefore, the series is divided into many small self-contained volumes to allow the clinician to purchase only those applicable to one's practice. As skills grow and new areas are approached additional titles can be added to form a complete library of surgical manuals.

The authors of each manual are noted experts within dermatologic surgery with a background in teaching. We are all very excited to participate in this new series as we are committed to dermatologic surgery and its role within our specialty. We hope you find these manuals of great practical use.

Roy C. Grekin, M.D.
Chief of Dermatologic Surgery
Department of Dermatology
University of California, San Francisco
School of Medicine
San Francisco, California

PREFACE

Dermatologic surgery is a rapidly growing subspecialty within dermatology. A standard part of the residency training program in dermatology now includes the surgical management of skin malignancy, wound healing, and local flap and graft reconstructive surgery.

This manual is designed to provide a practical approach to the techniques of skin grafting. The book includes detailed discussions of donor and recipient site considerations, the factors that must be considered in planning the repair of specific defects, specific instrumentation required for the various grafting procedures, postoperative wound care, and the complications particular to skin grafting. Besides the basic techniques of split and full thickness skin grafting, more complex techniques such as skin graft meshing and composite grafting for nasal alar and eyebrow reconstruction are included.

This manual was originally intended for the dermatology resident in training and for the surgical dermatologist. However, because of the paucity of manuals on skin grafting, this book should be valuable to surgeons in training in any other specialty that deals with the repair of cutaneous defects. While the techniques discussed certainly may be performed under general anesthesia, this manual emphasizes their performance in the ambulatory setting.

John W. Skouge, M.D.

CONTENTS

4. Composite Grafting / 65

Index /77

1

Basics of Skin Grafting

Skin grafting has been used as a reconstructive tool for centuries. At various times, each component of the skin (i.e., the epidermis, dermis, and subcutaneous fat) has been transplanted alone or in combination to achieve some reconstructive end. Split thickness and full thickness skin grafts are widely used in reconstructive surgery today, although epidermal, dermal, and dermal-fat grafts have had proponents at various times in the past. While there may be some specific indications for these other types of grafts, for the purposes of this manual, the term skin grafting will refer only to full thickness and split thickness grafts.

Full thickness and split thickness grafts are generally given very specific definitions. A split thickness graft is defined as consisting of epidermis and a partial thickness of dermis, while a full thickness graft is defined as consisting of epidermis and the complete thickness of dermis. Although these definitions cover the broad outlines of split and full thickness grafts, subtle variations of each graft type exist which require further explanation. At times, a full thickness graft may contain fragments of adipose tissue on its undersurface or, conversely, may be defatted to such an extent that some of the deep dermis is removed, creating, in essence, a thick split thickness graft. Moreover, split thickness grafts are actually subclassified as thin, medium, or thick, according to the amount of dermis included in the graft. Often, these split thickness grafts have very different indications as well as different ultimate aesthetic and functional results.

The surgical techniques of skin grafting can be readily learned and, with practice, significant skill in the harvesting and placement of grafts can be attained. As with any procedure, the key to ultimate success depends not only on the perfection of the technique itself but also on the proper application of the procedure. Therefore it is important to place the role of skin grafts into perspective with the other options for repair of cutaneous defects.

In this manual, the various techniques for harvesting of both split thickness and full thickness skin grafts are discussed. In addition, the preparation necessary for grafting, cosmetic and functional considerations referable to the donor and grafted site, and complications of grafting are explored.

WOUND HEALING CONSIDERATIONS

Unlike a flap, which carries with it its own blood supply through the flap pedicle, a skin graft is separated completely from its vascular system at the time of harvesting. The survival of the graft entirely depends on the nutritional support of the recipient wound.

For any graft to survive, three conditions must exist. First, the graft itself must have the potential for survival after removal. Second, the recipient site must be able to provide the necessary vascular supply for long-term survival of the graft. Third, during the interval between placement of the graft onto the recipient bed and vascular attachment and healing, the local environment must be favorable enough for attachment to occur.

Graft Quality

For a graft to have the potential for surviving the grafting process, the graft must consist of healthy tissue. It is important that the graft not be compromised, as can occur with radiation exposure. The graft must then be handled carefully during harvesting and processing, so it remains viable.

Period Between Graft Placement and Graft Take

Small vessel reattachment begins 48 to 96 hours after grafting. Before this time, the bed provides support to the graft by the process of imbibition, a passive uptake of nutrients by the graft. Special precautions must be taken when grafting to prevent anything from interfering with the reattachment of the graft to the wound bed. Factors that can interfere with attachment of the graft include infection, hematoma or seroma formation, and movement of the graft over the wound bed.

Quality of the Recipient Site

A wound without adequate vascular supply will not support a graft. Adequate vascular supply is necessary even for a thin split thickness graft that seems to require only marginal nutritional support. There are local, regional, and systemic factors that produce a decreased vascular supply at the junction of the wound bed and the undersurface of the graft. These compromising factors can act alone or in combination to produce graft failure. It is best to anticipate these problems and adjust the reconstruction accordingly.

Local factors include nonviable tissue in the wound, such as crushed and burned material or foreign bodies. Irradiated tissue and excessive fibrosis at the base of the defect have inherently decreased vascular supplies. Exposed bone, cartilage, or tendon (without periosteum, perichondrium, and peritenon) are relatively avascular. Regional factors include venous or arterial insufficiency or sickle cell disease. Systemic disorders can have equally negative effects. Examples of systemic factors include rheumatoid arthritis, systemic lupus erythematosus, other autoimmune diseases, and the microvascular changes that accompany diabetes. The appropriate history and physical examination will help uncover such conditions before surgery.

Ionizing radiation exposure produces fibrosis and vascular damage that makes surgical repair difficult. Local skin flaps that arise from radiation-damaged tissue may not have sufficient vascularity to survive, and the decreased blood supply in the wound base may not permit adequate survival of full thickness grafts. Such a wound may require split thickness repair or repair with a distant flap.

The vasoconstriction induced by nicotine has been clearly shown to decrease survival of skin flaps. A similar risk probably exists for grafts. Patients should be strongly discouraged from smoking during the perioperative period.

Among the most compromised wounds are lower leg ulcers. Usually, these ulcers are caused by a compromised vascular supply, either local or systemic. The most common underlying causes include venous and arterial insufficiency and sickle cell anemia. The problem is further complicated by the ulcer's location on the lower leg, which is highly susceptible to traumatic injury. Furthermore, such chronic ulcers are usually bacterially contaminated. This combination of factors makes treatment more difficult.

The ideal tissue for repair of a compromised wound is a flap. The flap would not depend on the marginal blood supply of the wound but would carry with it its own blood supply. The full thickness of dermis with attached adipose tissue would serve as a cushion to protect against injury. Unfortunately, such tissue is rarely available or practical. When surgical treatment is indicated, a graft may be the only reasonable repair option possible. Because of the vascular compromise, a thin split thickness graft is often the only tissue that may survive.

2

Split Thickness
Skin Grafting

DEFINITION

A split thickness skin graft may be defined as a fragment or sheet of skin that consists of epidermis and a portion of the underlying dermis. Split thickness grafts are subdivided into thin, medium, and thick grafts (Table 2-1), according to the amount of dermis included in the graft (Fig. 2-1). Thickness is usually measured in thousandths of an inch rather than in millimeters.

The medium thickness skin graft serves as a compromise between the advantages and disadvantages of thick versus thin split thickness grafts. In fact, medium thickness grafts are most frequently used by surgeons. Understanding the differences between the various subtypes of split thickness grafts, however, permits the surgeon the option of choosing a thin or thick graft, if the circumstances are appropriate.

A thin graft has a greater potential for survival than does a thick graft. Anatomically, dermal blood vessels arborize as they rise within the dermis. A thin graft, which is cut in a high plane in the dermis, has a finer capillary network exposed on its cut undersurface. In theory, this permits more rapid and diffuse connection between the vessels of the graft and those of the recipient bed. A thin graft also has less total tissue that requires revascularization. The increased probability that a thin graft will survive is particularly important when grafting a wound where the vascular supply is, for some reason, compromised.

Thin grafts are, however, more fragile and susceptible to traumatic injury than thick grafts. The greater amount of dermis contained in a thick graft acts like a cushion that helps prevent breakdown of the graft in the event of minor injury. This cushioning effect is particularly beneficial when the graft is placed on exposed surfaces such as the pretibial leg, where injury is frequent.

Table 2-1. Classification of Split Thickness
Grafts (Inches)

Thin	.008–.012
Medium	.012–.018
Thick	.018–.030

Although a thick split thickness graft results in a deeper injury to the donor site, it often has the potential for creating a somewhat better cosmetic result than a thin split graft. The factors that give skin its texture and color include the thickness of dermis, its vascular system, and the various adnexal structures contained in the dermis. Since a thick graft contains more of these elements, a better ultimate cosmetic result can be expected. Thick split thickness grafts do take a longer time to heal, and the risks of postoperative morbidity are greater.

Generally, split thickness grafts heal with a relatively poor cosmetic result as compared with full thickness reconstructions. Occasionally, a surprisingly good color and texture match is obtained. However, the usual split thickness graft heals with a shiny, atrophic, and pale appearance that contrasts markedly with the appearance of the surrounding skin. Although thicker split thickness grafts can result in a better appearance than thin grafts, the improvement is modest at best. Subsequently, split thickness grafts should be viewed as functional rather than cosmetic repairs.

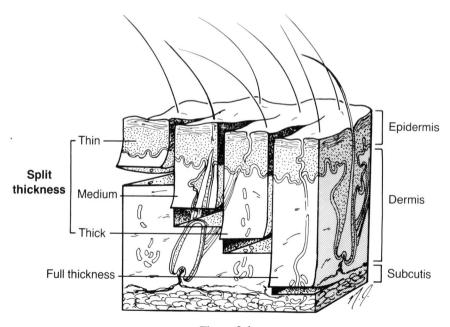

Figure 2-1

INDICATIONS

There are no absolute indications for split thickness grafts. In dermatologic surgery, they are used most often to repair defects created after skin cancer removal and to attempt repair of leg ulcers of various types. The relative indications for split thickness grafts are listed below.

As a repair for defects that are too large for coverage with a flap or full thickness graft

As temporary coverage after removal of a malignancy when it is important to observe the area for recurrence

As temporary coverage to prevent infection when a delayed reconstruction is expected

To provide backing for a flap when reconstructing full thickness defects

To provide coverage for wounds that are compromised when full thickness grafts would not survive

Large Defects

Split thickness grafts are often used for repair of defects that are either too large or located in an area that is impractical to repair with a full thickness graft or a local or distant flap. When making this decision, it is important to consider the cosmetic needs, age, and health of the patient. When aesthetic considerations dominate, it may be necessary to undertake the extraordinary measures needed to transfer a large amount of full thickness skin, whether that be via extensive dissection for a large local flap, a distant or microvascular flap, or a large full thickness graft.

Observation for Recurrence of Cancer

A split thickness graft may be used for reconstruction after skin cancer removal when the quality of the margins is questionable. Covering such a wound with full thickness skin may result in delayed recognition of a deep tumor recurrence. However, the thin covering provided by a split thickness graft creates a window that allows the surgeon to observe the area, thereby permitting earlier recognition of a recurrence. These concerns may override the cosmetic considerations relating to split thickness graft placement. At a later time, often 6 months to 1 year after grafting (when the risk of recurrence is diminished), the graft can be removed and a more definitive and cosmetic surgery can be performed if desired. Interestingly, many patients refuse reconstruction, because they have grown accustomed to the appearance of the split thickness graft.

As Posterior Lining to Flaps

Split thickness grafts can be used as the posterior lining for flaps used to repair through-and-through defects. This technique is probably used most commonly for flap reconstruction of full thickness defects involving the ala nasi. A split thickness graft placed on the back of the flap will provide the internal lining of the nose, while the flap itself covers the external surface.

DONOR SITE CONSIDERATIONS

Once the decision has been made to repair a wound with a split thickness graft and the proper graft thickness has been selected, the donor site must be chosen. It should always be borne in mind that a second, iatrogenic wound is created by the surgeon when grafting. Surprisingly, the donor wound is frequently more problematic for the patient than is the grafted site. It can be the source of significant postoperative morbidity and may result in an unsightly donor site scar.

When choosing a donor site, the thickness of the donor skin must be considered. Skin thickness varies with anatomic location and age. In general, a child's skin is thinner than an adult's and a woman's skin is thinner than a man's. In addition, the skin atrophies with advancing age and with debilitating disease. Awareness of these factors may prevent deeper harvesting than intended.

Other factors that must be considered when choosing a donor site include the following:

Cosmesis of the resultant donor scar
Type of instrument used to harvest the graft
Ease of postoperative donor site care
Color and texture match of the graft to the recipient area

Virtually any anatomic site can serve as a donor site for grafting. When the appearance of the donor site scar is of prime importance, the buttock serves as an excellent donor since the scar can usually be hidden completely beneath a bathing suit. The postoperative care of these wounds is more difficult, but the priority of scar placement may be a primary consideration for some patients.

Frequently, the particular area of the body chosen for the donor site is determined by the technical requirements of the instrument used to harvest the graft. The power-driven Brown and Padgett dermatomes and the large freehand knives, which are used to harvest larger grafts, require a flat surface with underlying support for grafting. Preferred sites include the anterior, lateral, or medial thighs, the buttock, and the abdomen (Fig. 2-2). Large grafts taken from the thigh are harvested with the long axis of the graft oriented along the long axis of the limb. Small grafts harvested freehand or with the Davol unit can be taken from nearly any location without considering the orientation (Fig. 2-3).

The ease of postoperative wound care of the donor site may dictate the site chosen for harvesting. This is especially true for elderly and debilitated patients, who may be operated on in the ambulatory setting and who are

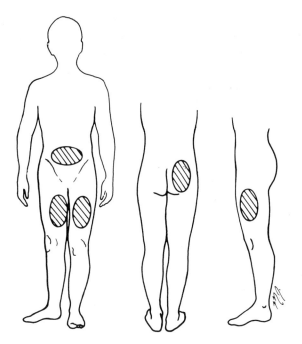

Figure 2-2

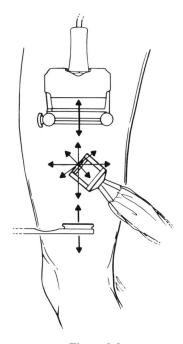

Figure 2-3

cared for by family. In these situations, the practicality of wound care may take precedence over the cosmesis of the resulting donor scar. The anterior and lateral thigh offer many advantages as the preferred donor site in such cases. These sites are readily accessible to the surgeon, and wound dressings are easily applied. These wounds are also easily cared for by family and patient. In addition, wounds in this location permit relatively free ambulation by the patient because they do not interfere with sitting, bending, or sleeping.

For facial reconstruction, some surgeons prefer skin taken from above the shoulders, the so-called blush zone. A split thickness graft taken from this area will retain some capacity to blush, resulting in an overall superior cosmetic result. For this purpose, the scalp is sometimes utilized as a donor source. Since hair follicles are not included in the graft but are left behind, hair is not transferred with the graft. Scalp hair will then regrow, concealing the donor scar. A significant disadvantage to selecting the scalp as a donor site is that the shaved scalp leaves the patient cosmetically compromised for a significant time while hair regrows. In addition, the small benefit derived by transferring skin with blush capacity does not outweigh the marginal cosmetic result typical of split thickness grafts.

Taking all of these factors into consideration, most large grafts are harvested from the anterior, lateral, or medial thigh, because harvesting and wound care is most convenient. When cosmetic considerations are primary, the buttock serves as the donor site of choice. Small grafts are taken from the inner or outer upper arm or thigh.

PREPARATION FOR GRAFTING

Preparation of the donor site involves shaving the skin, prepping with one of the surgical scrubs, and draping. If Opsite is used as the postoperative dressing for the donor defect (see the section on donor site care), the entire area that will be covered by the dressing should be shaved.

The skin must be kept taut around the donor site during harvesting, no matter which skin grafting system is used. Since several hands are usually needed to accomplish adequate skin tension, split grafting requires an assistant. Without applying the proper tension, the skin will bunch and fold in front of the instrument, thereby inhibiting grafting altogether or, at the very least, creating an irregularly cut graft.

A skin lubricant is also necessary, for ensuring easy movement of the cutting instrument. The traditional lubricant used in skin grafting has been sterile mineral oil. Concerns about oil droplets remaining beneath the transferred graft and resulting in foreign body reactions have been unfounded. While sterile mineral oil is an excellent lubricant, any of the sterile water-soluble surgical lubricants work very well. They are easily obtained and eliminate the need to maintain sterile mineral oil in the surgical area.

Measuring the Defect

Accurate measurement of the defect is critical to prevent cutting a graft that is too small for repair of the defect. Most defects are relatively flat and a ruler will usually suffice for accurate measurement. However, using a straight ruler for complicated defects that cover convexities or concavities, such as auricular defects, will result in inaccuracies. For these types of defects, a template is used to more accurately measure the surface area. The use of a template is discussed on page 52. It is important to note that all defects have a vertical component to their sidewalls. For particularly deep wounds, the surface area involved may be considerable. This additional surface area must be included in the measurement of the defect to ensure accuracy of measurement.

Sterile Technique

Sterile technique is particularly important when grafting. Since a graft consists of devitalized tissue, the risk of infection at the grafted site is greater than when tissue that carries its own vascular supply is transferred. Coincidentally, the risk of infection at the donor site is probably very low, due in part to the superficial nature of the injury created.

Antibiotic coverage is not required for all grafting procedures. Antibiotics are recommended when wounds have been left open several hours or when contamination of the wound is assumed. The most common bacteria in surgical wounds are *Streptococcus* and coagulase-positive *Staphlococcus*. Pseudomonas is of concern particularly around the ear. Chronic leg ulcers present a difficult problem since they are usually contaminated by bacteria. Gram-positive or gram-negative organisms may be found, and often several different organisms will grow out. Proper culture and sensitivity studies are needed routinely in anticipation of grafting such wounds.

Anesthesia

Choice of anesthesia depends on the health of the patient, surgical indications, and patient comfort. General and regional anesthesia are rarely indicated for split thickness grafting in the setting of dermatologic surgery. Even large grafts can usually be harvested safely under strict local anesthesia.

Local anesthesia with 1 percent lidocaine with epinephrine 1 : 100,000 is most often used. However, lower concentrations of each agent can be equally effective. The pain of injection can be lessened with the use of a 1 inch, 30 g needle. Buffering of the anesthetic solution from the packaged pH of 4.0 to a more physiologic level can also decrease the pain of injection. One ml of 8.4 percent sodium bicarbonate per 10 ml of local anesthetic will raise the pH to nearly physiologic level. Once buffered, the anesthetic should not be stored because the epinephrine breaks down rapidly, resulting in reduced efficacy.

Epinephrine is contraindicated in patients who are β-blocked or who are taking antidepressants. In addition, it is advisable to avoid its use in individuals who have significant hypertension or heart disease, for whom the additional adrenergic stimulus may be problematic. Even without the vasoconstrictive benefit of the epinephrine, there is only minimal and self-limited bleeding.

Intradermal, rather than subcutaneous, infiltration of the anesthetic most efficiently produces anesthesia. Since the injury created by harvesting involves only the dermis, a subcutaneous injection is unnecessary. Intradermal injection causes slightly more discomfort during infiltration, but produces almost immediate anesthesia while requiring only the minimum amount of anesthetic to be injected. Occasionally, a strictly subcutaneous injection will produce incomplete anesthesia of the overlying skin.

Surgical Set-Up

In addition to the particular harvesting tool needed for split thickness grafting, the following instruments are recommended for placement on the surgical tray.

Sterile surgical marking pen
Syringe with 1 inch, 30 g needle
Scalpel handle and #15 blade
Toothed tissue forceps
Iris scissors (serrated if available)
Needle holder
Suture or stapler as indicated
Petri dish with sterile saline
Mosquito hemostats × 2

The scalpel included on the tray is sometimes needed for final separation of the graft from the donor site. Iris scissors must be on the tray. The serrations on the scissor blade give the surgeon greater control when trimming slippery split thickness grafts. The Petri dish is used to hold the graft on saline-moistened gauze after harvesting, until it is placed onto the recipient site. The hemostats are beneficial when using the Brown or Padgett dermatomes and serve to hold the graft, while it is being cut, so as to avoid bunching. Holding the graft also permits the surgeon to monitor the thickness and quality of the graft during harvesting.

GRAFTING INSTRUMENTS

A wide variety of instruments for harvesting split thickness grafts has been developed over the years. Grafting instruments are classified into freehand, drum, and electric dermatomes (Table 2-2). In this section, the more commonly used instruments are discussed, along with the advantages and disad-

Table 2-2. Split Thickness Grafting
Instruments: Classification

Freehand
Razor blade
#15 Surgical blade
Weck knife
Drum
Electric
Davol dermatome
Brown dermatome
Padgett dermatome

vantages of each. The surgeon should be proficient in the use of at least two techniques, one for cutting large grafts and one for harvesting small ones. Mastering two techniques permits the surgeon to deal comfortably with wounds of various sizes (Table 2-3).

Freehand Dermatomes

Freehand refers to cutting grafts with a hand-held knife. All freehand systems cut grafts manually, with the surgeon using a back-and-forth sawing motion. Freehand instruments include the standard single- or double-edged razor blade, the #15 Bard-Parker surgical blade, and any of the grafting knives, such as the Weck knife and the Humby knife.

Drum Dermatomes

Before the advent of electric dermatomes, drum dermatomes were widely used for cutting large grafts. These instruments are cumbersome to assemble and difficult, even dangerous for the surgeon to handle. By and large, they have been replaced by the simpler, Brown and Padgett electric dermatomes, which are simpler to use, safe, and reliable. The particular use of the drum dermatome will not be discussed.

Table 2-3. Split Thickness Grafting
Instruments: Graft Size Produced

Small	Large
Freehand	
Razor blade	Weck knife
#15 Surgical blade	
Electric	
Davol dermatome	Brown dermatome
	Padgett dermatome

Electric Dermatomes

Electric dermatomes perform the back-and-forth cutting action for the surgeon. These tools have greatly simplified split thickness grafting and generally produce better quality grafts, more reliably. There are three commonly used electric dermatomes: the Davol, Brown, and Padgett units. The Davol unit cuts only small grafts. The Brown and Padgett units are the workhorses for harvesting large split grafts. Because all are used commonly for skin grafting, each will be discussed, along with its particular advantages and disadvantages.

HARVESTING

Freehand Grafting

Razor Blade

The most basic freehand grafting instrument is the double-edged razor blade that is used for shaving. The razor blade comes from the manufacturer clean but not sterile. It cannot be steam-autoclaved, because it will rust. Instead, it must be gas-sterilized. Since gas-sterilization can be an inconvenience, some surgeons sterilize the blade at the time of surgery by placing it in Sidex or an equivalent antiseptic solution. The blade may be used whole or split in half. Only small, irregularly edged grafts that are 2 to 3 cm wide can be cut with this system.

TECHNIQUE

Step 1. The donor site is prepped, shaved, draped, and anesthesized. A thin coating of sterile lubricant is placed on the skin and the blade.

Step 2. The razor blade is held between the thumb and index or third finger and is placed exactly parallel to the skin surface.

Step 3. Applying only a gentle back-and-forth motion and minimal downward pressure, the blade is advanced through the skin at the proper depth. The extreme sharpness of the blade permits cutting of the graft with only minimal tension applied to the surrounding skin (Fig. 2-4).

The thickness of the graft can be estimated. Grafts that are translucent are generally less that 15-thousandths of an inch thick. Grafts become opaque beyond this thickness.

PITFALLS

Grafts harvested by razor blade are usually irregular in thickness and rather small. The razor blade is flexible and very sharp. As a result, caution is required to prevent a deeper injury than planned.

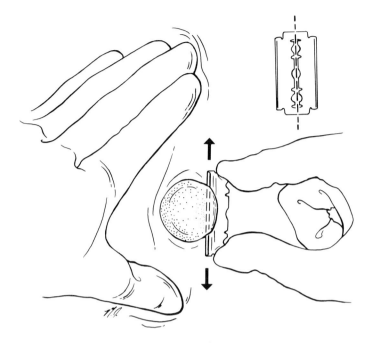

Figure 2-4

Bard-Parker #15 Blade

The #15 blade can be used to harvest small- to medium-sized grafts. This technique requires more practice than other techniques, but is very useful for simple skin grafting. It permits cutting a graft with the exact dimensions required for the wound. All other instruments cut square or rectangular grafts, whose corners must be sacrificed to accommodate the circular or oval, irregularly shaped defects most often encountered.

TECHNIQUE

Step 1. The donor site is chosen. Almost any location can serve as the donor site, although flat or convex surfaces work best. The lateral upper arm or thigh is often used. The site is then marked, prepped, and infiltrated with anesthetic. The exact size of the graft needed is marked.

Step 2. The blade is attached to a scalpel handle. With the scalpel held perpendicular to the skin, the tip of the blade gently scores the skin around the perimeter of the graft (Fig. 2-5). The incision is carried only into the superficial papillary dermis, when capillary bleeding is first noted. The depth of the scoring is so superficial that the weight of the scalpel itself is sufficient to achieve the desired depth. The scoring permits the blade to track along the scored line during harvesting.

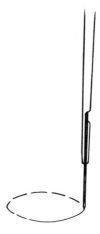

Figure 2-5

Step 3. A minimal amount of surgical lubricant is applied to the skin.

Step 4. The assistant applies multidirectional traction around the donor site while the surgeon applies countertraction with the noncutting hand. Adequate traction is critical in successful grafting when using a #15 blade.

Step 5. With the blade held parallel to the skin, the tip of the blade is inserted into one side of the scored perimeter.

Step 6. The blade is gently pulled from one side of the graft to the other, slowly increasing the amount of graft cut with each pass. Only minimal forward pressure is needed. Note that the blade will naturally follow the scored perimeter (Fig. 2-6).

Step 7. When grafting comes to completion, pick-ups will be needed to hold the free margin of the graft, to prevent it from folding onto itself and interfering with the last few cuts necessary to free the graft (Fig. 2-7).

PITFALLS

If the graft becomes too thin, or if the blade cuts through the graft (called button-holing), harvesting is stopped from this access and begun from another edge. Any small hole can simply be left alone or sutured at the time of graft closure. With practice, a 3 cm diameter split thickness graft can be harvested in several minutes.

Weck Knife

The Weck knife is designed to harvest larger grafts. It comes with a handle, disposable blades, and several templates that control graft thickness. There are other freehand knife systems available, but the Weck is the most commonly used.

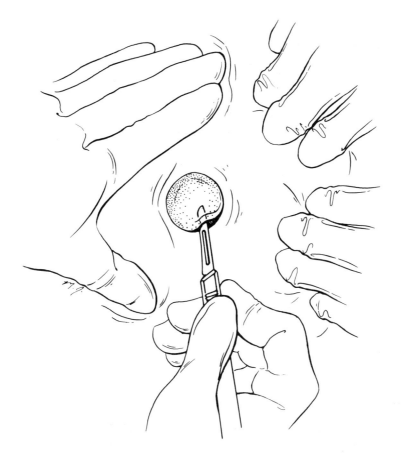

Figure 2-6

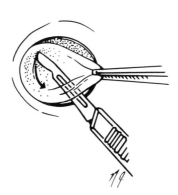

Figure 2-7

TECHNIQUE

Step 1. The Weck blade is slid onto the handle and the template is attached.

Step 2. The usual preparations are made for grafting as described above. The assistant provides tension across the skin for grafting.

Step 3. The blade is placed parallel to the skin. Using a back-and-forth sawing motion, the knife is advanced through the skin. Moderate downward pressure and only mild forward pressure are required. Graft thickness is determined by the pressure applied or predetermined by the template. The sawing motion of the knife is the major force in the actual cutting of the graft. To complete harvesting, the downward pressure on the skin can be eased, and several more back-and-forth strokes will separate the graft. Alternatively, grafting can be stopped and the graft separated with scissors or scalpel blade (Fig. 2-8).

PITFALLS

The mechanical nature of the grafting system will create saw-toothed edges on the graft. These edges are generally sacrificed before placement of the graft. Therefore, the remaining graft is slightly narrower than might be expected. It is important to anticipate this, so that there is adequate graft for covering the defect.

Pinch Grafts

Surgeons have used pinch grafts for many years. Because the technique is a simple one, pinch grafting has had many advocates. Unfortunately, the cosmetic results are often unacceptable. The technique will be described briefly, merely to demonstrate the significant disadvantages of the technique. Pinch grafts have been recommended for use on wounds that are draining significantly. The spaces between the small graft fragments permit drainage to leak out without lifting the grafts from the wound surface.

TECHNIQUE

Step 1. The donor site is prepped and anesthetized. The instruments needed for pinch grafting are basic: only iris scissors and pick-ups.

Step 2. The donor skin is grasped (pinched) by the pick-ups and gently lifted. The iris scissors serve to snip off the small fragment of lifted skin (Fig. 2-9).

Step 3. The graft, which is usually less than 1 cm in diameter, is placed onto the recipient wound. Multiple grafts may be harvested for large defects and are placed a small distance apart from each other. The spaces between the grafts heal by epithelialization.

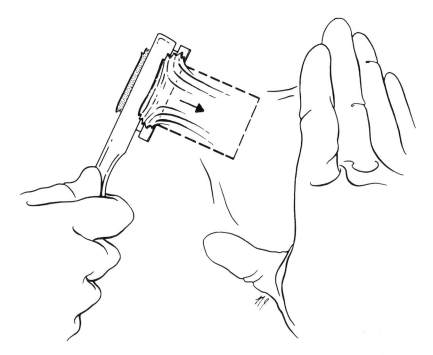

Figure 2-8

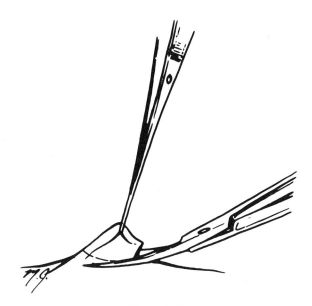

Figure 2-9

PITFALLS

The simplicity of the technique can be alluring, especially for those with little surgical background, but there are several disadvantages. The grafts created by pinch grafting are not of even thickness. The graft edge only consists of epidermis. The amount of dermis progressively increases from the edge to the center of the graft. Therefore, the healed grafts appear like multiple small hillocks at the recipient site, while the donor site is left pock-marked.

Alternative techniques for harvesting small grafts, described in this manual, are equally simple to master and result in superior quality grafts. These methods should relegate pinch grafting to a position of mere historic interest.

Electric Dermatomes

Davol Dermatome

The Davol-Simon dermatome is a battery-powered unit that was developed to cut small split thickness grafts. Its advantages are simple design and use. The specifications of the instrument are as follows.

1. Graft width is fixed at 3.0 cm.
2. Only relatively short grafts can be harvested, since the quality of the blade will not permit harvesting long lengths of graft.
3. The thickness of graft is fixed at 15 thousandths of an inch.

The Davol handle is portable, has an internal rechargeable battery, and cannot be sterilized. The handle is used with a disposable kit that contains a single-use, sterile grafting head with blade attached and a sterile plastic bag with twist.

TECHNIQUE

Step 1. The contents of the disposable kit, which are sterile, are placed on a sterile tray (Fig. 2-10).

Step 2. The surgeon, wearing sterile gloves, holds the sterile plastic bag as an assistant carefully drops the nonsterile handle into it (Fig. 2-11). The twist secures the end of the bag and creates the sterilized unit necessary. The cutting head is clicked into place over the bag onto the end of the handle (Fig. 2-12). The unit is now ready for use.

Step 3. The donor site is prepared in the standard manner. The assistant applies the necessary tension on the skin around the donor site.

Step 4. The cutting side of the dermatome is placed on the skin, applying only moderate downward pressure. The unit is turned on. Mild forward pressure with the Davol dermatome will harvest the graft (Fig. 2-13).

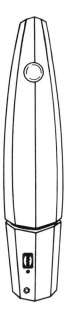
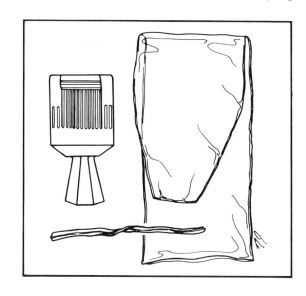

Figure 2-10

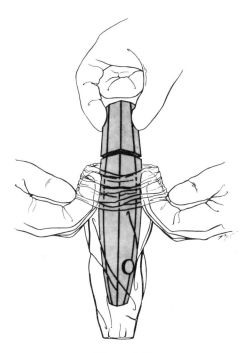

Figure 2-11

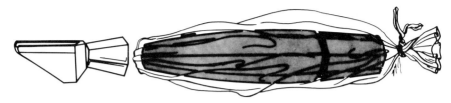

Figure 2-12

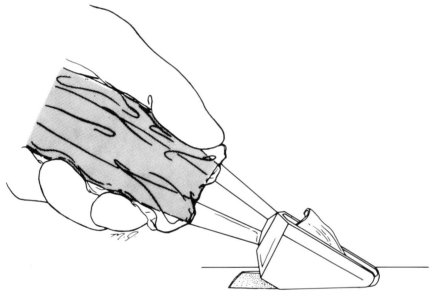

Figure 2-13

PITFALLS

The only major problem that can arise relates to the battery. If the unit has not been adequately charged, or if the battery is weak, there may not be sufficient power to complete grafting.

Brown and Padgett Electric Dermatomes

The Brown and Padgett electric dermatomes have become the standard instruments for harvesting large split thickness grafts. Both instruments cut grafts of various thicknesses and widths easily and predictably. These instruments are so reliable that they have eliminated the need for the large freehand grafting knives.

There are important differences between the Brown and the Padgett units.

1. The Brown dermatome is steam-autoclavable, while the Padgett unit must be gas-sterilized. Because large gas sterilization units are relatively inaccessible to nonhospital-based surgeons, most office-based practitioners use the Brown unit. However, special arrangements can be made with a hospital so that the Padgett can be adequately sterilized.

2. The Padgett unit is sturdier and has fewer moving parts than does the Brown. Consequently, it requires fewer repairs. Because of its increased reliability, the Padgett unit is more often found in hospital operating rooms, where its sturdy nature is required for longevity and where gas sterilization is readily available. In the office setting, where few staff handle the instrument, the Brown dermatome can be handled gently and can be maintained with relatively little maintenance for long periods.

3. The Brown unit permits precise adjustments of graft width, whereas the Padgett, on the other hand, comes with three templates from which to choose. The templates measure 2, 4, and 6 inches in width. Some waste of skin can be expected when using the Padgett dermatome, resulting in a somewhat larger donor defect and scar. However, the graft thickness settings are more reliable with the Padgett unit. The Brown unit must be calibrated before each use. While this is an added nuisance, the calibration is easily performed and is only a minor inconvenience.

BROWN DERMATOME TECHNIQUE

Step 1. The donor site is prepared for grafting, marked, and infiltrated with anesthetic.

Step 2. The Brown dermatome must be assembled. In addition to the instruments on the surgical tray described above, the following components of the dermatome are needed: dermatome and unsterilized motor; disposable dermatome blade; and sterile wrench. The three screws on the back of the dermatome that secure the blade must be maximally loosened. The disposable blade is then placed over the three projecting rivets, and it is checked to be certain the blade is flush with the casing. The screws are then tightened with the sterile wrench included with the dermatome (Fig. 2-14).

Step 3. The graft thickness settings must be calibrated before use. The thickness dials on the Brown unit are marked in thousandths of an inch. Both dials must be moved simultaneously, or there can be only 5-thousandths of an inch difference between the two settings at any one time. Straying from these parameters may put the unit out of alignment. The calibration for graft thickness is performed in the following manner.

A. Both dials are set at a thickness setting of zero.

B. The unit is turned over and examined to be sure that the cutting portion of the blade is in intimate contact with the casing.

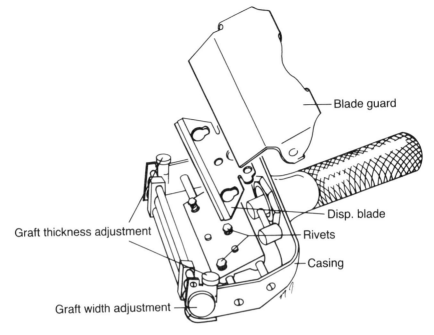

Blade guard

Disp. blade

Graft thickness adjustment

Rivets

Casing

Graft width adjustment

Figure 2-14

C. The graft thickness dial is set at 15 thousandths of an inch. Conveniently, a Bard-Parker #15 blade is approximately 15 thousandths of an inch thick at its cutting edge. This setting on the unit should just permit the placement of the scalpel blade between the dermatome blade and the casing on the undersurface of the unit.

D. With these two settings confirmed, the desired thickness can be set and harvesting may proceed.

Step 4. The graft width setting is then made. The dial is located on the side of the unit and permits the surgeon to set the exact width of graft needed.

Step 5. The skin and dermatome blade are lightly coated with lubricant. Only a very thin layer is necessary.

Step 6. The assistant applies traction on the skin, away from the surgeon. The surgeon holds the dermatome with one hand, and the other is placed behind the unit and pulled toward him, providing counter-tension.

Step 7. The flat cutting portion of the dermatome is placed on the skin to prepare for harvesting. Applying moderate downward and slight forward pressure, the foot pedal is pressed to start the dermatome. A graft of equal thickness will result.

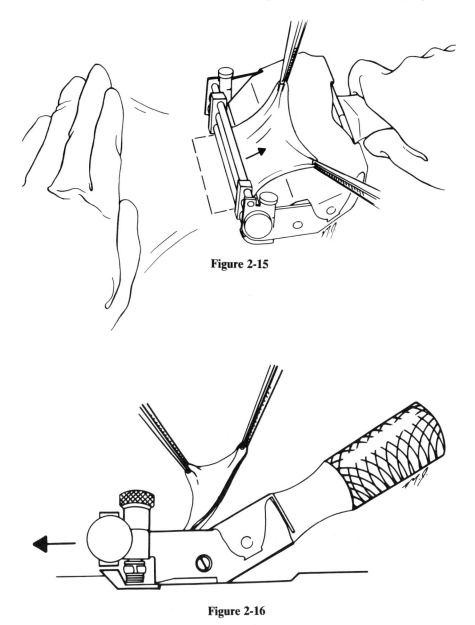

Figure 2-15

Figure 2-16

Step 8. Forward progress is halted and the unit is stopped when the graft
begins to appear above the blade. Without lifting the dermatome
from the skin, the assistant grasps the two corners of the graft with
hemostats. While harvesting, the graft is lifted away from the unit,
permitting the surgeon to monitor the thickness and quality of the
graft (Fig. 2-15). *Note:* It is critical that the cutting undersurface be

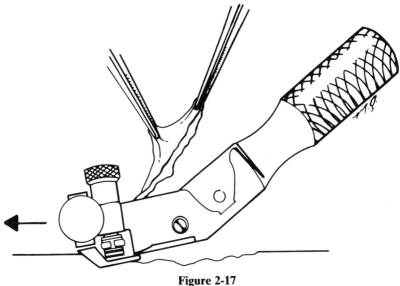

Figure 2-17

exactly flat with the skin (Fig. 2-16). If the front tip of the dermatome is pressed down, an irregularly thick graft will result (Fig.
2-17).

Step 9. When harvesting is complete, the front (cutting) end of the dermatome is lifted, as if it were an airplane taking off. This action will
almost always separate the graft from the donor site. If it does not
separate them, the dermatome must be stopped immediately or the
graft will be damaged. The graft can be manually separated from the
donor using the surgical blade.

Step 10. The graft is placed on the sterile saline-soaked gauze in the Petri dish
until ready for placement onto the recipient site.

PITFALLS OF THE BROWN DERMATOME

Stopping the unit to allow the assistant to attach the hemostats may leave a
visible line on the graft at that point, which may be cosmetically noticeable
upon healing. If the surgeon is confident of the functioning of the dermatome,
this step can be eliminated. The graft will simply bunch up on the back of the
blade during harvesting. Elimination of this step speeds up the harvesting
process but does not permit the surgeon to monitor the grafting process. The
advantages of monitoring the harvesting process may override the slight

cosmetic defect that results from the pause taken during grafting. If an uneven graft is being harvested, one or both thickness settings can be reset, and grafting resumed.

PADGETT DERMATOME TECHNIQUE

The Padgett unit includes the following:

Dermatome
Disposable blade
Templates for setting graft width
Sterilizable screw driver

Assembly of the Padgett dermatome is straightforward. The blade is set into position on the undersurface of the dermatome casing. The template of appropriate width is chosen and placed on top of the blade. Both are then secured with the screw driver (Fig. 2-18).

Step 1. The usual preparations for grafting are made.

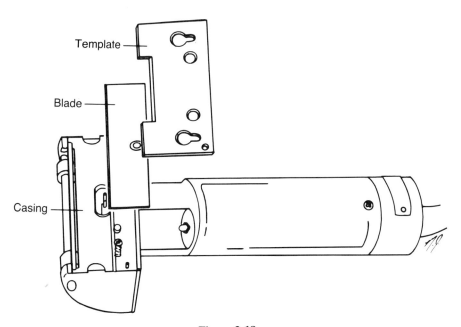

Figure 2-18

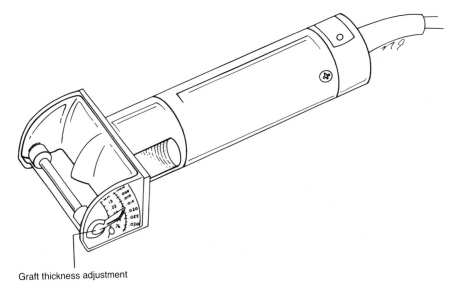

Graft thickness adjustment

Figure 2-19

Step 2. Graft thickness is selected by adjusting the single dial on the side of the dermatome (Fig. 2-19). The setting is very accurate and no calibration is necessary.

Step 3. The skin and blade are lubricated. The appropriate tension is applied to the skin around the donor site by the assistant and the surgeon. The flat cutting surface of the dermatome is placed onto the skin and, with only moderate downward and minimal forward pressure applied to the unit, the graft is harvested. The technique is essentially the same as for the Brown dermatome.

SECURING THE GRAFT

If a grafted site could be kept completely immobile, and if infection or hematoma or seroma formation did not occur, a graft could simply be draped over a defect without suture or support and the graft would survive. Unfortunately, since virtually all dermatologic surgery patients are ambulatory, it is imperative that the graft be meticulously secured and efforts made to prevent occurrence of those factors that may interfere with the ultimate survival of the graft.

Virtually all grafts should be secured with a combination of suture or staple and support dressings, to ensure that the graft is connected to both the surrounding skin and the wound floor. Securing the perimeter of the graft only to the skin surrounding the defect is normally not sufficient for graft take. Since the nutritional support for the graft comes from the tissues below rather than by percolation across the graft from the edges, the graft must also be held securely to the base of the defect. The graft is held to the wound base by pressure dressings or centrally placed basting sutures.

Securing the Perimeter of the Graft

The perimeter of the graft can be secured with suture or staples. The precise approximation of skin edges that is necessary for suturing full thickness skin is not as critical with a split thickness graft, nor is the meticulous suturing technique as important.

If the graft overlaps slightly onto adjacent skin, it will simply slough, without adverse effect on the ultimate result. The separation of the nonviable skin may take several weeks or more. During the intervening period, however, these rough edges can be uncomfortable for the patient because they can catch on clothes and dressings.

Simple, interrupted sutures or a running stitch can be used in securing the graft perimeter. For small grafts, interrupted stitches may suffice. For large grafts, an over-and-under running stitch is more efficient and is entirely adequate for closure. Placing several anchoring, interrupted sutures at various points around the perimeter of the graft is recommended to provide added security to the running stitch. These interrupted sutures help position and orient the graft during placement. In addition, anchoring the running stitch to these interrupted stitches will prevent complete unraveling in the event that the sutures break in the postoperative period.

The caliber of suture material used depends on the thickness of the skin surrounding the defect and the stresses that the area will encounter during the postoperative period. Ideally, there should be no tension on the closure. Therefore, 6-0 suture should be adequate to secure most grafts. Occasionally, 5-0 suture will be required. Whatever gauge suture material is used for the running stitch, material that is one size larger is generally recommended for the anchoring stitches. For example, when 6-0 is used for the running stitch, 5-0 is used for the anchors. No specific suture material is recommended. Any of the nonabsorbable synthetic sutures work well, although one of the rapidly absorbing, chromic gut sutures, which dissolve in 5 to 10 days, can greatly simplify suture removal.

Perimeter Sutures

TECHNIQUE

Step 1. The graft is trimmed and placed over the defect.

Step 2. The 5-0 interrupted, anchoring sutures are placed at several locations around the defect. The sutures are left slightly long so they may be secured by the running stitch. For most grafts, a suture is placed at each of four quadrants (Fig. 2-20).

Step 3. The 6-0 running stitch is started immediately adjacent to one of the anchoring sutures. The over-and-over stitch is secured to each of the anchoring sutures without cutting the stitch and starting over (Fig. 2-21). When the running stitch has been secured to the last anchoring suture, the perimeter of the graft is secure.

Hints: Recall that most harvesting systems produce grafts that are rectangular in shape and larger than the defect. It is important to cut the excess graft carefully to prevent overtrimming. One method of preventing overtrimming is to place the anchoring stitches before the graft is trimmed, which permits more accurate orientation of the graft over the defect (Fig. 2-22). Alternatively, excess graft can be trimmed one quadrant at a time, placing the running suture immediately following the trimming of each section of graft. Either of these two methods helps prevent miscalculations and excessive trimming of the graft.

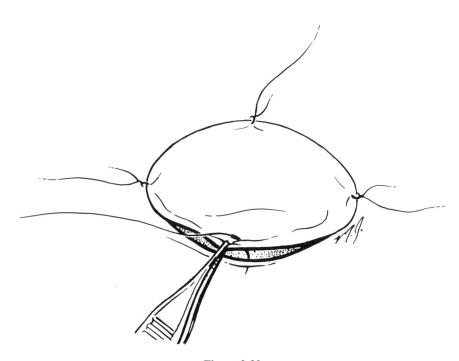

Figure 2-20

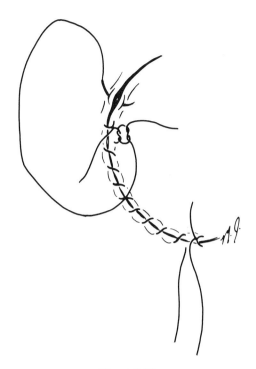

Figure 2-21

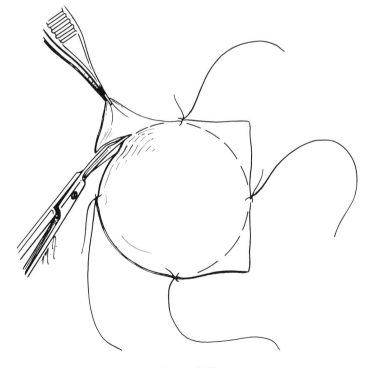

Figure 2-22

Stapling

Skin staples can be useful when grafting on relatively thick or immobile skin such as the scalp, forehead, or back. The primary difficulty with staples is that, when they are closed into place, they tend to gather graft skin with them, pulling the graft toward the edge of the defect (Fig. 2-23). This gathering effect stretches the graft and places increased tension on its center.

Securing the Central Portion of the Graft

After the perimeter is secured, the remainder of the graft must be kept in contact with the wound bed. Attaching the graft to the wound bed is accomplished with either suture or support dressing.

Basting Sutures

Basting stitches can be placed to hold the graft to the wound bed. Various suturing techniques have been described. Individual, interrupted 5-0 or 6-0 sutures are placed through the graft and a small portion of the defect below (Fig. 2-24). Multiple basting sutures can also be used.

A running basting stitch, described by Glogau, can be used to secure a large graft to the wound bed quickly (Fig. 2-25). In addition to holding the graft

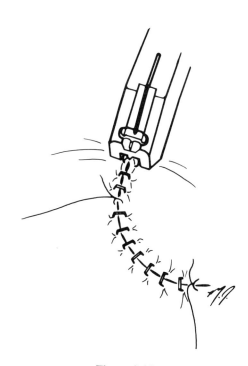

Figure 2-23

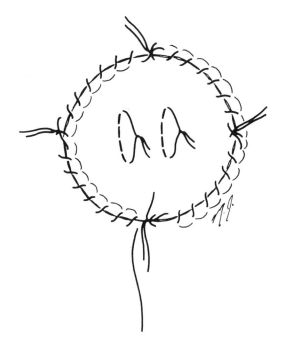

Figure 2-24

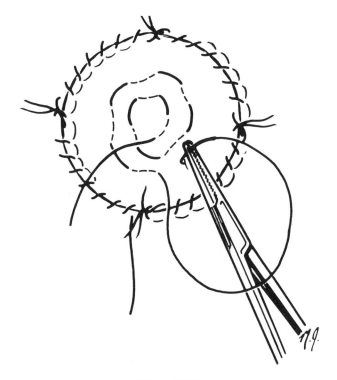

Figure 2-25

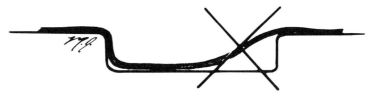

Figure 2-26

to the base, these stitches will tend to loculate any hematoma or seroma that may form, thereby limiting dissection of the fluid between the graft and the bed.

Whichever technique is used for securing the graft, it is important to remember that most wounds have a vertical dimension as well as the obvious horizontal dimension. The graft must be secured to the defect sidewalls. A tightly pulled skin graft will tend to tent over these concave areas, resulting in loss of that portion of the graft (Fig. 2-26).

Dressings

The choice of dressing depends on many factors, including the location of the grafted site, the degree of ambulation of the patient, and the need to observe the graft during healing.

A simple dressing, whose purpose is to protect the graft from environmental contamination, may be adequate for some grafts, such as small grafts, grafts that have been adequately secured with suture, or grafts placed over convex surfaces, such as the forehead. In addition, a dressing of this type may be preferred if the wound needs to be observed for complications during the postoperative period. Such a dressing consists of an antibiotic ointment for the suture line, covered by an nonstick layer, such as Telfa or Adaptic.

Dressings have also been designed to provide continuous pressure and immobilize the grafted site until healing is complete. The tie-over dressing is frequently used for these purposes.

TIE-OVER DRESSING TECHNIQUE

The tie-over dressing is intended to provide constant, even pressure on the graft during the immediate postoperative period. It is secured in place with sutures tied over the dressing and is usually not disturbed until suture removal.

Step 1. The graft is secured to the wound as described above. Central basting sutures may or may not be indicated.

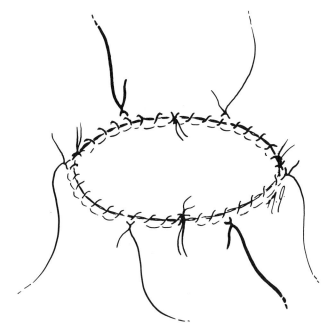

Figure 2-27

Step 2. The sutures used to tie over the dressing are placed. In order to provide even pressure across the dressing, sutures are placed in pairs, opposite each other across the graft. Interrupted sutures, 3-0 to 5-0, are recommended. These are placed in the skin, immediately adjacent to the graft edge, and are left long so they can be used to tie over the dressing (Fig. 2-27). The suture ends may be held with hemostats to keep them out of the surgical field until needed. Small grafts may require only four sutures. Larger grafts may need six or more.

Step 3. A layered dressing is applied. A light coating of antibiotic ointment placed at the perimeter keeps the suture line soft, and may facilitate removal of the dressing when the sutures are removed. A nonstick layer is then placed. N-terface, Telfa, Adaptic, or other nonstick materials are adequate.

Step 4. The last layer serves to mold the dressing to the contours of the wound below. A variety of materials has been described for this use. Sterile cotton balls soaked in sterile saline or water are easy to use. They are individually rung out and packed over the defect (Fig. 2-28). When the cotton balls dry, they will harden, creating a firm, exact mold of the defect below.

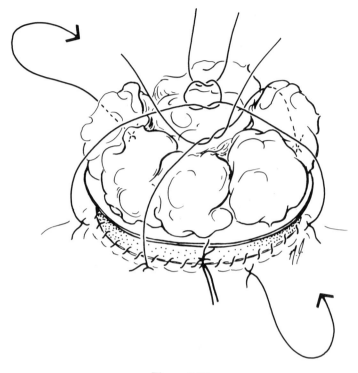

Figure 2-28

Step 5. The dressing is secured with the tie-over sutures. Each stitch is tied to its paired partner on the other side of the graft. Then each pair is tied to the others for added security (Fig. 2-29).

   The dressing is now complete and, in general, will not be removed until the time of suture removal. If desired, a cosmetic gauze dressing can be placed over this.

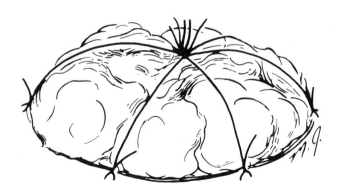

Figure 2-29

ADVANTAGES OF TIE-OVER DRESSING

There are many advantages to the tie-over dressing:

1. It completely isolates the wound from the environment.
2. It provides constant, even pressure on the graft, which helps to keep the graft in contact with the wound bed and assists in the prevention of hematoma or seroma.
3. It immobilizes the graft.
4. It minimizes daily wound care for the patient. If exudate does form around the edge, the patient is encouraged to gently clean with peroxide and reapply a small amount of antibiotic ointment.

PITFALLS OF TIE-OVER DRESSING

The only significant disadvantage of the tie-over dressing is that the status of the graft cannot be monitored without destroying the integrity of the dressing. If a complication, such as hematoma, seroma, or infection, were to occur, these problems might go unnoticed, or recognition might be delayed until that affected portion of the graft is lost. In an effort to prevent this problem, some have suggested placing the sutures at the time of surgery, but not securing the tie-over dressing until one day afterward, when the risk of bleeding is reduced. Others have suggested removing the dressing at 24 to 48 hours, so the graft can be examined, then replacing the dressing with a more traditional one. These variations offer occasional advantages in selected patients, but for the most part, they also serve to complicate the surgery and the postoperative wound care.

If a tie-over dressing is to be employed, sterile technique also must be employed, and the potential complications of using the dressing must be analyzed, in order to optimize its advantages. In skin cancer work, the advantages of the tie-over dressing usually outweigh the disadvantages, especially in the ambulatory setting.

DONOR SITE CARE

The grafting process creates a second wound, the donor defect, for which we must also provide care. While it may seem secondary in importance to the wound that has been grafted, these donor wounds are usually more difficult to treat, and usually cause more pain and symptoms for the patient than the grafted site itself. Proper postoperative donor site management can greatly improve the patient's comfort and speed the healing process.

Over the years, various methods have been advocated for the postoperative care of split thickness graft donor wounds. However, the development of the semipermeable membranes has most significantly improved our management of such wounds. These dressings, like Opsite, offer many advantages over traditional dressings. When these dressings are left in place throughout the healing period, the pain, which was almost incapacitating with traditional dressings, is significantly reduced. The dressings allow the serosanguinous drainage that occurs to be collected beneath them. The fluid then acts to keep the wound moist, which decreases healing time. The transparent nature of the dressing permits the wound to be seen during the healing process. The dressing also simplifies wound care for the patient and family.

The large amount of serosanguinous fluid produced by donor site wounds can be problematic when it collects beneath the Opsite dressing or other semipermeable membrane. When the fluid builds up, it has the tendency to track beneath the dressing. When its path is complete, the fluid drains out all at once, which can be frightening for the patient and family if they are not forewarned. They should be told that the greatest amount of fluid is produced in the first two days after surgery and that it decreases each day after.

The following instructions, if followed, will aid in the handling of the donor site.

1. The entire area to be covered by the Opsite is shaved. If possible, this should be done at the time of grafting.

2. After grafting, the skin surface around the wound should be cleaned of all blood, serum, and surgical soap, all of which decrease the adherence of the Opsite.

3. A thin coat of tincture of Benzoin or other skin adhesive is applied to the area that the Opsite will cover. Of all the adhesives available, Benzoin and Mastisol seem to work best in this setting. It must be allowed to dry before the Opsite is applied. Avoid applying the adhesive to the wound itself.

4. Opsite is awkward because it readily sticks to itself. Therefore, its application requires two people. With an assistant, the Opsite dressing is placed over the wound, using the largest sheet practicable. The dressing should extend at least 1 inch from the donor site edges. The larger size provides a broader area for serum to collect without leaking. For best results, the Opsite must be applied without wrinkles, which only serve to provide an avenue for leakage of the fluid. The green, nonstick edges of the dressing are then carefully trimmed away.

5. For extra support, a 2 inch wide strip of tape is placed around the perimeter of the Opsite. Microfoam tape from 3-M works especially well for this purpose. A gauze dressing is then placed at dependent sites around the Opsite to collect the leakage of serum, should it occur.

Placement of this dressing seems complicated, but actually it takes only 5 minutes to apply and is well worth the effort required.

If possible, the dressing should be changed in 1 or 2 days. The amount of fluid that collects after this time is usually small enough that the dressing can then be left in place until the wound has completely healed. At the time of the dressing change, an additional gauze dressing is usually not necessary and the patient can then shower normally.

There are times the patient cannot return for the dressing change. Unfortunately, we have found it virtually impossible to teach family to apply a new Opsite dressing at home without great difficulty. If there are problems with the dressing at home, it can be removed and a more traditional dressing can be applied, but this alternative is discouraged.

It is important to forewarn the patient and family that leakage around the dressing may occur at home, so they will not fear that the wound has suddenly begun to bleed heavily. In such an event, the area can be cleaned and a piece of skin tape applied over the site at the edge where the fluid leaked out. Since the dressing is no longer completely intact, leakage will continue at this site. A gauze dressing placed at this location will collect the drainage. The Opsite dressing can be left in place. Since leakage tends to occur at the most dependent part of the Opsite dressing, reinforcement with gauze, when the dressing is originally placed, is recommended.

If desired, the fluid can be drained without removal of the Opsite dressing. A needle inserted through the dressing into the fluid collection can be used to suction out most of the fluid. The hole can be simply patched with a small postage stamp-sized piece of additional Opsite dressing. It is important to note that infection beneath an Opsite dressing used for donor site care has never been reported, even when it has been left in place for several weeks.

When it is time to remove the Opsite dressing, the patient is instructed to stand in the shower or sit in the tub, and very slowly peel it off. If the fluid beneath it has dried, the Opsite dressing will occasionally adhere to the newly epithelialized skin and small portions of the skin may be removed with the dressing.

POSTOPERATIVE EXPECTATIONS

Most of the problems encountered during the postoperative period relate to patient comfort during healing and the problems of graft survival. Barring intervening problems, this process should last less than two weeks.

Patient comfort is critical during this period. Discomfort, generating primarily from the donor site, can usually be alleviated with acetaminophen or a mild narcotic analgesic. Infection is always a concern. Surgical wounds that are promptly grafted do not necessarily require antibiotic support. Contaminated wounds require appropriate antibiotic coverage. Patient education is probably the single most important factor in avoiding significant problems during this time.

Ultimately, the goal when grafting is 100 percent survival of the graft. Whenever this goal is not reached, it is important to evaluate all aspects of the procedure, including the technique used, environment of the wound, health of the patient, and any complicating factors that prevented the goal from being attained.

Under ideal circumstances, the graft should "take" in 3 to 5 days. At this early stage, however, the new vascular connections are fragile and easily disrupted. Therefore, the sutures and dressings are generally left in place for a slightly longer time, for added protection. At the time of suture removal, the graft color should be pink to violaceous. Any vesicle formation or clear-cut necrosis noted at this point indicates that a portion of the graft has been lost. Large vesicles should be carefully opened and drained if there is concern that the fluid might dissect beneath adjacent viable graft. Otherwise, they may be left alone. Vesicles serve as sterile dressings and reepithelialization will progress beneath them. Except in the setting of infection, no debridement is necessary.

After suture removal, usually no dressing is necessary, except as a cosmetic cover and protection from external trauma. A light covering is usually recommended and desired by the patient.

MESH GRAFTING

The process of graft meshing involves the placement of regular arrays of slits in the graft. The primary purpose of meshing is to permit the graft to expand in an accordion-like fashion so that the graft can cover a larger surface area. This technique is particularly advantageous in situations where skin is in short supply, such as in patients who are severely burned.

Mesh grafting is rarely indicated in the dermatologic surgery setting. Wounds are only rarely large enough to require the increased coverage attainable with a meshed graft. There is usually abundant donor skin available for most grafting purposes without having to resort to meshing.

Mesh grafts can be useful, however, for defects that are draining significant amounts of fluid or for those that are bacterially contaminated. The slits in the graft permit wound drainage to escape freely, thereby preventing fluid build-up beneath the graft.

There are several disadvantages of graft meshing. The spaces between the slivers of graft remain open and must heal by epithelialization. This prolongs the healing time of the graft. After healing, the graft usually retains the criss-cross pattern produced by the mesher, which can be cosmetically unsightly. These disadvantages give meshed grafts a limited usefulness for repair of defects on the face.

The Zimmer skin mesher is a simple machine used for meshing. The system consists of the mesher and detachable crank, both of which are stainless steel and can be sterilized. In addition, sterile, single-use, grooved, plastic carriers are included. The groove pattern on the carrier defines the size of the resultant holes to be placed in the graft. Carriers are designed to permit expansion to one and one-half, three, or six times the original area of the graft.

TECHNIQUE

Step 1. The mesh cutter and crank, as well as the plastic carrier, are placed

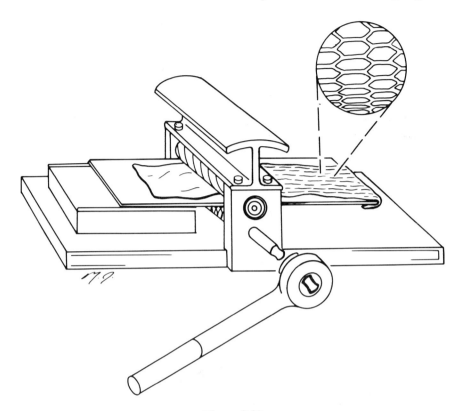

Figure 2-30

on a sterile field. The heaviness of the unit and the manual nature of the procedure require that the unit be placed on a firm table top rather than on a Mayo stand. The crank is attached to the mesher (Fig. 2-30).

Step 2. The graft, usually large in size, is placed dermal side down onto the ridged surface of the plastic carrier. The leading edge of the graft must be draped slightly over the carrier edge, so that it will not be pushed away from the meshing surfaces of the cutter (Fig. 2-30).

Step 3. The plastic carrier and graft are introduced between the two cutting cylinders of the mesh cutter (Fig. 2-31). As the hand crank is turned, the carrier and graft move through the cutter (Fig. 2-32). Once meshed, the graft is fragile and difficult to handle, and should be transported from the mesher to the defect while still on the carrier.

Step 4. The graft can simply be draped onto the defect or secured into place in the usual manner. Some form of support dressing is required to hold the meshed graft in place. Loosely placed basting sutures can be helpful to hold the central portion of the graft to the wound bed.

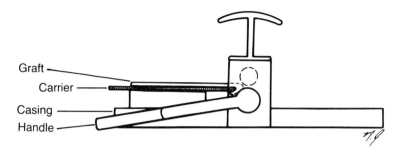

Graft
Carrier
Casing
Handle

Figure 2-31

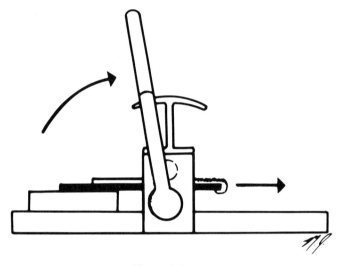

Figure 2-32

COMPLICATIONS

Complications of split thickness grafting are divided into early and late complications and are summarized in Table 2-4. Early complications are those resulting in a graft's failure to survive. These are secondary to technical errors, complications during the immediate postoperative period, and inadequacies inherent in the initial defect that was grafted.

Early Complications

Technical

Though it may seem trivial to mention, it is important not to place the graft upside-down when grafting. It is usually easy to distinguish between the two sides of the split thickness graft, because the dermal side is shiny, while the epidermal surface appears dull. However, the distinction between the two sides can be blurred when a lubricant is used, because a lubricant can lend a somewhat glistening appearance to the epidermal surface. A simple trick is to remember that a split thickness graft always curls onto itself and always curls toward the dermal side.

Hematoma/Seroma Prevention

Problems with hematoma and seroma formation must be anticipated so that the adverse effects can be prevented. First, a decision must be made as to whether the wound is graftable. A wound that is draining profusely is probably not ready for grafting and requires further preparation before a graft can be attempted. Despite these precautions, hematoma or seroma formation can occasionally occur, even in cases where wounds are graftable.

There are several precautions that can be taken to deal with small to moderate amounts of fluid build-up. Meticulous hemostasis and an adequate pressure dressing are critical factors in preventing these problems. In addition, if bleeding or oozing in the immediate postoperative period is expected, the patient should be encouraged to elevate the grafted wound and minimize movement-related activities.

There are several techniques that can be employed during surgery to minimize the build-up of fluid beneath the graft. While grafting, small slits, like those made when baking a pie, can be cut through the graft. Single or multiple cuts can be placed if necessary. The slits permit drainage and prevent build-up underneath the graft. Dependent areas and concavities are most prone to fluid collection. In extreme cases, a meshed graft can be used (see the earlier section on meshed grafts).

Table 2-4. Complications of Split
Thickness Grafts

Early—failure in graft survival
   Technical considerations
      Upside-down graft
      Inadequate immobilization
   Postoperative considerations
      Hematoma and seroma formation
      Infection
      Movement
   Inadequate recipient site (compromised)
      Inadequate blood supply
      Circulatory incompetence
      Systemic disease
Late—aesthetic and functional deficits

If hematoma/seroma formation is noted within 48 hours after grafting, the fluid can be drained without interfering with graft survival. A gauze pad may be rolled over the affected portion of the graft, toward the nearest edge, to extract it. This technique may, however, disrupt some early vascular connections. Often, an easier approach is simply to cut a small, slit directly over the collection, to drain the fluid.

Infection

Strict sterile technique is the best prevention against infection. Fresh surgical wounds frequently can be grafted without antibiotic coverage. Wounds that have remained open for hours or contaminated wounds may require coverage with the appropriate antibiotic(s). Thin split thickness grafts will survive over some contaminated wounds. Chronic ulcers require preparation as well as frequent wound culture and sensitivity studies so that the appropriate antibiotic coverage is given. If the risk of infection is high, a tie-over dressing may be contraindicated, as early signs of infection may go unnoticed and appropriate treatment may not be undertaken.

Movement

Movement-related complications are often preventable at the time of surgery with proper suturing technique and choice of support dressings. Ambulation after surgery may lead to movement-related graft failure. Therefore, this possibility must be anticipated, if at all possible, so that adequate instructions can be given to the patient and family.

Late Complications

Aesthetic Considerations

It is best to consider a split thickness graft a functional, rather than cosmetic, repair. Occasionally, they will heal with a surprisingly good match of color and texture. The usual expectation, however, is that the color and texture of the healed graft will contrast markedly with the surrounding adjacent skin. Normally, at least some final depression to the healed wound can be expected, if the original defect is depressed. Wound contraction is to be expected with a split thickness graft. The contraction generally involves the tissue below the graft, and may create a wavy and uneven appearance in the overlying graft.

Pigmentary changes can be a considerable long-term problem with split thickness grafts. Specific color changes are difficult to predict. Only on occasion, does the color seem to match reasonably well. Such a match tends to occur in very fair-complected patients in whom the graft also heals with hypopigmentation. In addition, the absence of adnexal structures that characterize split thickness grafts creates a xerotic surface and a build-up of keratinous debris and scale, which gives the graft a dark appearance.

Functional Considerations

Split thickness grafts contract far more than full thickness grafts. It is estimated that there may be as much as a 70 percent contraction of split thickness graft sites. The forces of contraction can be very powerful, resulting in joint contractures when a graft is placed on or near a joint. Of particular concern to the dermatologic surgeon is the issue of contraction of grafts on the face, particularly near the free margins of the vermilion, the nasal ala, or the eyelid (especially the lower). With rare exception, wound contraction forces will overpower the forces of the underlying musculature, resulting in pulling of these important structures away from their normal anatomic locations. When this occurs on the lower eyelid, adjacent cheek, or nose, ectropion formation can be the result. Distortion of the vermilion and retraction of the ala nasae, although not usually of functional concern, can result in significant cosmetic deformity.

Graft fragility may exist when split thickness grafts are placed on defects with little underlying soft tissue for support, or in settings of marginal vascular supply, as these locations are susceptible to traumatic injury. This problem is seen commonly when grafts have been placed over vascular insufficiency ulcers on the lower legs, pressure points (such as in treatment of decubitus ulcers), or directly on top of perichondrium or periosteum. These problems may be chronic and difficult to treat.

3

Full Thickness
Skin Grafting

DEFINITION

A full thickness skin graft consists of epidermis and the full thickness of dermis. Occasionally, some fat may be included on the undersurface of the graft (Fig. 3-1).

INDICATIONS

Full thickness grafts can be used almost anywhere on the face. They are most valuable for repairing small- to medium-sized defects when full thick-

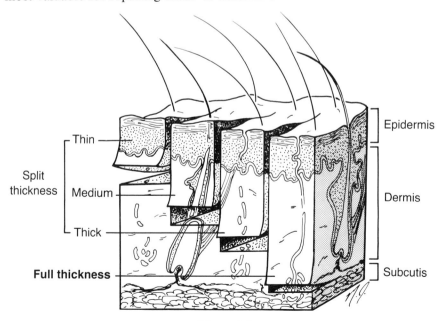

Figure 3-1

ness skin is necessary and a flap is not available or practicable. When the decision has been made to use a graft, a full thickness graft is chosen over a split thickness graft when the ultimate cosmetic and/or functional result is the predominant consideration.

A full thickness graft may be indicated over a local flap for repair of a defect for any of these reasons:

1. There is not sufficient adjacent skin for development of a local flap.
2. A flap will result in sufficient scarring or deformity that the graft offers a better cosmetic result.
3. A distant or microvascular flap is impractical.

A full thickness graft is preferred over a split thickness graft when wound contraction will result in functional deformity, or when the ultimate cosmetic result is preferred over that produced by the split thickness graft.

Specific Facial Defects for which Full Thickness Grafts May Be Useful

Full thickness grafts are most often used in locations where there is little redundant skin for development of a local flap. Such sites include the nasal tip and ala, the lower and (to a lesser extent) the upper eyelids, the auricular helix, and the upper lip. Full thickness grafts are also useful for repair of larger defects on the temple and forehead when a local flap is impractical. They are occasionally used in other locations on the face, but most often there is adequate local tissue for flap reconstruction.

Nasal Tip

On the nasal tip, full thickness grafts are useful for defects involving skin or skin plus soft tissue. At this site, there is rarely skin available for side-to-side or local flap repair and forehead flap reconstruction may not be practical. A full thickness graft can produce an excellent cosmetic result in this location.

Nasal Ala

The skin of the ala is bound down, and therefore there is rarely adequate adjacent skin for local flap repair. Transposition flaps, especially nasolabial, rhombic, or bilobed, are useful for reconstruction of such defects. Since these flaps come from higher on the nose, movement generally results in distortion or ablation of the alar groove, which serves as the superior margin to the alar subunit. Wound contraction resulting from a split thickness graft or second intention healing on the ala will preferentially pull upward on the free margin of the alar rim, which can cause significant distortion. In addition, the color and texture match is frequently inadequate when a split thickness graft is used for repair, especially in patients with sebaceous skin. The healed site will usually take on a "tire patch" appearance. For these reasons, a full thickness graft may provide the best reconstructive choice for defects limited to the subunit of the ala.

Lower Eyelid

Functional concerns referable to the eye are of foremost importance when reconstructing the lower eyelid. The slightest amount of wound contraction may result in ectropion formation and corneal injury. Therefore, split thickness grafts and granulating wounds, both of which contract markedly, are only rarely acceptable repair options in this location. Local flap reconstructions are very useful for small defects when there is sufficient redundant eyelid skin. However, wound contraction can occur with these repairs, which can pull down the eyelid margin. Full thickness grafts are frequently preferred for repair of such defects, as wound contraction can be minimized or prevented. Placement of a graft that is 150 to 200 percent of the defect size is recommended.

Auricular Defects

Full thickness grafts are frequently employed for auricular defects, again because of the limited local skin available for flap repair. Underlying intact cartilage usually prevents wound contraction, so that a split thickness graft or second intention healing can be employed. The color deficit associated with a split thickness graft on the ear must always be considered.

Temple and Forehead

Moderate-sized defects on the temple and forehead are not infrequent sites for full thickness graft repair because of a relative lack of adjacent tissue available for local flap movement. In these areas, a combined reconstruction using a partial flap repair along with a full thickness graft can give excellent results.

DONOR SITE CONSIDERATIONS

Because the full thickness of dermis is included in a full thickness graft, the vascular pattern and adnexal structures normally present in the dermis remain relatively undamaged after transfer. The color and textural properties produced by these dermal elements remain after the donor skin has been transferred (referred to as "donor dominance"). This characteristic of grafted full thickness skin permits the surgeon to examine various potential donor sites and choose the site that most closely matches the skin surrounding the defect to be grafted. This is in marked contrast to split thickness grafts, in which most of these characteristics are lost after grafting.

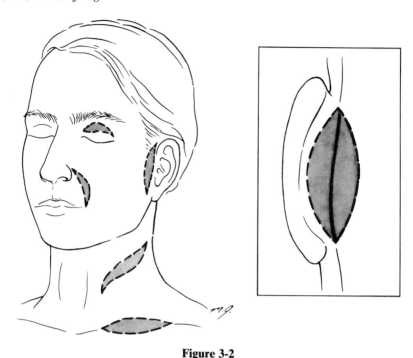

Figure 3-2

For facial defects, most full thickness grafts are taken from above the shoulders. Grafts taken from this so-called blush zone have a better chance of matching the textural and color features of facial skin. There are a number of factors that must be considered when choosing the donor site. These include:

1. The depth of the defect
2. The size of graft needed
3. The color and texture of the donor skin
4. The quality of the vascular supply of the recipient defect

Figure 3-2 illustrates the most commonly used donor sites for full thickness grafting. These sites are used because

1. They offer the best potential color and texture for facial defects.
2. There is usually sufficient redundant skin available.
3. The donor scar can be relatively easily hidden.

Postauricular Skin

The area of the postauricular ear and adjacent scalp is the most commonly used donor source for full thickness grafts. A relatively large supply of full thickness skin is available for harvesting and the resultant scar can be easily hidden. The major disadvantage of this site is the somewhat poorer color and texture match for some facial defects. Postauricular skin is relatively photo-protected in contrast to facial skin. As a result, this skin usually does not have the solar lentigines and elastotic changes that characterize severely sun-damaged facial skin. In addition, postauricular skin has fewer adnexal structures, seen as fewer pores. This is often in marked contrast to the skin of the central face, particularly the distal nose, where the skin is frequently very sebaceous and porous. Of secondary importance, the postauricular donor defect is often painful during the immediate postoperative period. Despite these negative attributes, the large supply of skin available and the ease of hiding the scar make this the prime donor source.

Postauricular grafts are useful for most facial defects. Because of the relative thinness of skin in this area, postauricular grafts often serve as the secondary source for eyelid defects (upper eyelid skin is the primary reservoir). The thinness of the skin also makes the postauricular site ideal for repair of auricular defects.

Preauricular Skin

The preauricular cheek can serve as the donor for small full thickness grafts. This site offers some advantages over the postauricular area as a donor site. The skin is usually thicker, has been sun-exposed and often provides a better color and texture match for the rest of the face. The resultant scar can be hidden in one of the prominent preauricular creases. This site is used more often in women. However, even in men, there is a thin strip of hairless skin between the sideburn and the ear. Unfortunately, excision of this skin in men places the sideburn closer to the ear, which can be cosmetically disturbing.

Supraclavicular Neck

The supraclavicular and the lateral neck serve as excellent donor sources of sun-damaged skin for full thickness grafts. Large grafts can be harvested and the color match can be quite good. In some, however, the skin may be thicker and more leathery than facial skin. Donor scars are more difficult to hide on the neck, especially in women who may be used to wearing clothes with lower neck lines.

Upper Eyelid Skin

When available, redundant upper eyelid skin (that which might be removed during blepharoplasty) serves as the ideal donor skin for lower eyelid and medial canthal defects. It is possible to use both upper lids in situations in which redundant skin on one lid is insufficient. In this situation, the two grafts can be sutured to each other.

Melolabial Fold

The melolabial fold may occasionally serve as an excellent source of sebaceous skin, especially when attempting to match nasal skin. It is often the only facial skin with characteristics similar to those of the distal nose. When planned carefully, with the ends of the fusiform placed exactly in the melolabial groove, the resultant scar can be completely hidden. Excision of one fold may produce some asymmetry, necessitating correction by removal of a like amount of skin from the other fold.

Other Donor Sites

Occasionally, skin below the neck is used as a donor for facial defects even though the color and texture match tends to less than ideal. Any location where there is thin, redundant skin, can serve as the donor for full thickness skin. The upper and inner arm, the volar forearm, the wrist, and the inguinal area can serve as donor skin for full thickness grafts.

PREPARATION FOR GRAFTING

The same preparations are necessary when reconstructing with a full thickness graft as with any facial reconstruction. Since a graft represents devitalized tissue and is more susceptible to infection, sterile technique is mandatory.

In the setting of dermatologic surgery, local anesthesia is usually sufficient for full thickness grafting, although the health and comfort of the patient and the specifics of the surgery will indicate the level of anesthesia used.

Measuring the Defect

It is obviously critical to measure the size of the defect accurately. On flat surfaces, the measurement can be performed simply with a ruler. For irregularly contoured surfaces, such as the convexity of the nasal tip or the concavity of the auricular concha, measuring with a straight ruler will result in inaccuracies. In these situations a template is used. A template used for measuring irregular defects consists of any flexible material that can be bent to conform to the defect. A sterile gauze, Telfa dressing, or piece of sterile aluminum foil will serve this purpose.

Measuring with a Gauze Template

TECHNIQUE

Step 1. A sterile 4 × 4 or 2 × 2 gauze serves as the template. The gauze is gently pressed into the defect to be grafted. The serosanguinous exudate in the wound will create an accurate bloody imprint on the gauze exactly matching the size of the defect (Fig. 3-3).

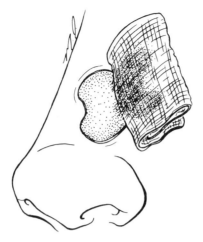

Figure 3-3

Step 2. The imprinted gauze is cut out.

Step 3. The template, *bloody side down,* is placed onto the skin of the proposed donor site and the outline of the template is drawn (Fig. 3-4). Always anticipate that the donor site will have to be closed. Most often, this closure is obtained using a fusiform design. Therefore, the proposed graft should be oriented to best fit into the relaxed

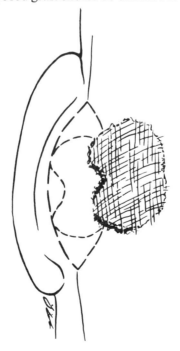

Figure 3-4

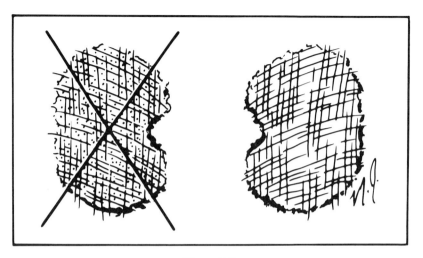

Figure 3-5

skin tension lines of the donor site, in anticipation of the needed repair. No matter what closure is anticipated, it is important to plan for that at this time. The template must *not* be placed upside-down, that is bloody side-up, when drawing the proposed graft, as this will create a mirror image of the defect (Fig. 3-5).

HARVESTING

TECHNIQUE

Step 1. The donor site is prepped and draped in the usual sterile fashion, and anesthetized. The outline of the graft is marked on the skin.

Step 2. With a #15 blade, the incision is carried through the skin and into the subcutaneous fat. Since the graft is always defatted after removal, the plane of dissection may be made at the level that will best facilitate donor site closure. Dissection in the plane of the superficial fat most often accomplishes this (Fig. 3-6). *Note:* The graft may be removed with the dog ears attached. This step can provide additional flexibility in case the defect has been improperly measured. However, excising the excess skin from the graft is more difficult after graft removal than before.

Step 3. The graft is placed on sterile, saline-soaked gauze in a Petri dish until needed.

DEFATTING THE GRAFT

The adipose tissue adherent to the undersurface of the graft is poorly vascularized. Since much of the nutritional support for the graft will come

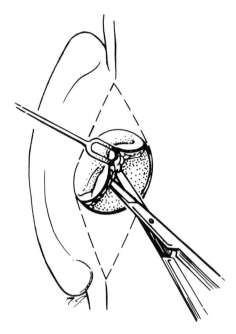

Figure 3-6

from the base of the defect, the fat must be removed from the graft so its deep dermal vessels will be in direct contact with the defect floor. This process of removing the fat is called defatting.

TECHNIQUE

Step 1. The graft, fat and dermal side up, is draped securely over the index or third finger of the nondominant hand and is supported by the thumb or a skin hook.

Step 2. Sharp, curved iris scissors, convex cutting edge toward the graft, are used for defatting. The fat is removed with small bites of the scissors, until a white, glistening dermal surface can be seen throughout. This represents a level at approximately the junction of the subcutis and the deep reticular dermis. The finger over which the graft is draped permits the surgeon to gauge the thickness of graft between the scissors and finger (Fig. 3-7). Care must be taken not to cut through the graft, "button holing," as even the smallest hole will result in a visible scar after healing. In such an event, the hole should be repaired with 6-0 suture at the time of closure.

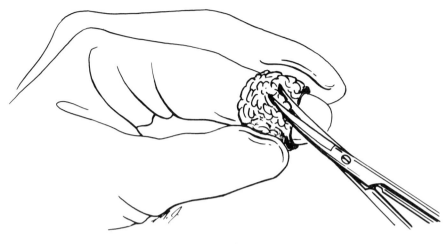

Figure 3-7

SECURING THE GRAFT

The same careful suturing technique is necessary when securing a full thickness graft as when suturing any full thickness skin. Proper approximation of the sutured edges is critical, since the ultimate cosmetic result often depends on the quality of suture technique used. This is in contrast to the technique required when suturing split thickness grafts, in which approximation of the graft edges to the wound edge need not be perfect.

Full thickness grafts, like split thickness grafts, are secured by one or all of these means:

Perimeter sutures
Basting sutures
Support dressings

Perimeter sutures are always needed. Basting sutures and support dressings are not always needed but are used when the central portions of the graft need additional support.

Perimeter Sutures

A 6-0 suture is used most often to secure facial grafts. Simple, interrupted stitches may be used. An over-and-over running stitch may be used, as long as approximation of the sutured edges is attained. It is advisable to secure a running stitch to several interrupted 5-0 sutures placed at various points around the perimeter. Attachment to secure points will prevent the suture from unraveling completely, were it to break during the postoperative period.

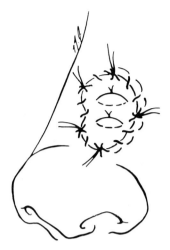

Figure 3-8

For small grafts, one of the rapidly dissolving mild chromic gut sutures used as the running suture can greatly simplify suture removal. These suture materials will dissolve in 5 to 10 days and therefore may obviate suture removal.

Basting Sutures

Single or multiple, 5-0 or 6-0 basting sutures can be placed to secure the central part of the graft. Because of the potential of such a stitch to produce a small scar, basting sutures are used less often than they are with split thickness grafts. They may be more useful, for securing large grafts, in providing extra support against movement, and for grafts placed on a concave defect where tenting of the graft is likely to occur (Fig. 3-8).

Support Dressings

Those factors that prevent the graft from attaching to the recipient bed will result in failure of the graft. The dressing that is placed over the graft can, therefore, mean the difference in graft take. When there is little chance the graft will shift during the healing period, a simple pressure dressing will suffice to hold the graft in place. An appropriate layered dressing includes a small amount of antibiotic ointment along the suture line, covered with a nonstick dressing such as Telfa, N-terface, or Vaseline gauze, which is then covered with an absorbent layer and secured with tape.

The tie-over dressing, described in Chapter 2, is frequently employed over full thickness grafts, as well as over split thickness grafts. As mentioned previously, this dressing is sutured over the graft, and is generally left in place until the the time of suture removal (Fig. 3-9).

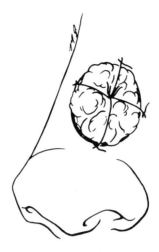

Figure 3-9

CLOSURE OF THE DONOR SITE

With full thickness grafting, an iatrogenically induced secondary wound and resultant scar are created at the donor site. It is, therefore, critical that the functional or cosmetic needs at the site to be grafted be considered more significant than the scar produced at the donor site. No matter how the donor site is closed, the resultant donor scar must be anticipated when planning the operation.

Closure of the donor defect requires the same planning as does the closure of any cutaneous defect. Most often, for small- and medium-sized grafts, the donor site defect is designed to conform to the shape of a fusiform and is closed in a side-to-side manner. However, when indicated, a local flap or split thickness graft may be used. Second intention healing can also be employed.

Since postauricular skin is used most often for facial full thickness grafts a few pertinent comments regarding this area are needed. A large amount of full thickness skin is available from the postauricular area. The skin covering the entire posterior aspect of the auricular concha can be used, if needed, along with an equivalent amount of skin from the adjacent scalp. A graft of 4 to 5 cm in diameter can be obtained in this manner, and the donor site can still be closed primarily. Approximation of the wound edges will, in the extreme, necessitate pulling back the ear (Fig. 3-10). Because of the strength of the underlying cartilage, however, this effect is only temporary and the ear will return to its original position. However, the postauricular sulcus will be shallower after the donor site has healed. Because of tension across the wound created by the auricular cartilage, buried, intradermal sutures are usually indicated. Vicryl or Dexon 4-0 or 5-0 sutures may be used. Without buried sutures, dehiscence is common with suture removal at 5 to 7 days.

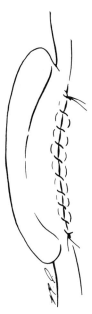

Figure 3-10

Sutures can be left in place for a longer period of time; however, the patient usually returns for suture removal at the grafted site at this time and it is convenient to remove all of the sutures at this time.

POSTOPERATIVE EXPECTATIONS

There is rarely significant postoperative discomfort at either the grafted or the donor site. A notable exception is the postauricular donor site, which can be the source of considerable discomfort. The reasons for pain at the postauricular site probably relate to the fact that the ear sticks out away from the head and is easily bumped and moved. Eyeglass placement and movement during sleep aggravate the discomfort. Nonetheless, acetaminophen is often adequate for pain relief and only rarely is a narcotic analgesic required.

The appearance of the graft at the time of suture removal may not indicate the extent of its viability. A graft may be pink, red, blue, or purple and remain completely viable. It is important to inform patients of this fact preoperatively. Occasionally, a graft will appear ominously black and necrotic and may certainly represent total loss of the graft. It may, however, reflect only a superficial loss of epidermis, or epidermis and papillary dermis, with viability of the deeper portions of the graft. A graft that has lost the epidermis and superficial dermis resembles the depth of injury induced by dermabrasion or a deep chemical peel. Such a wound heals slowly, by epithelialization, and a reasonable or even excellent cosmetic appearance can result. At the time of suture removal, it may be impossible to distinguish partial from full thickness dermal necrosis. *Therefore, eschars should not be debrided!* The patient and family should be reassured and the area watched carefully. In the event of full thickness loss of all or a portion of the graft, the undebrided graft will serve as a natural dressing, under which healing will progress. After several months, an assessment of the extent of the loss can be made and revisional surgery planned as necessary.

COMPLICATIONS

Complications relating to full thickness grafting relate to (1) the short-term problems of graft failure, and (2) the long-term functional and cosmetic problems.

Graft Failure

One hundred percent survival of full thickness grafts should be the expected outcome. Those factors that might interfere with graft survival must be anticipated so this result can be achieved. The most common interfering factors include infection, hematoma or seroma formation, and movement, as well as factors related to the quality of the recipient defect.

Infection

Infection after grafting on the face is rare. Nonetheless, sterile technique is particularly important. Antibiotics are not routinely used, but may be helpful in selected patients. Prevention of factors that may contribute to the risk of infection must also be avoided, especially hematoma or seroma formation, bacterial contamination of the graft or recipient site, and harsh handling of the graft due to poor surgical technique.

Hematoma and Seroma Formation

Meticulous hemostasis, proper wound dressing, and postoperative care will help decrease the risks of hematoma or seroma formation. The patient should be cautioned against vigorous activity, which may increase blood pressure and induce bleeding, especially in the first 48 hours after surgery. After grafting on the head and neck, patients are specifically instructed to avoid heavy lifting or bending over. During the first 24 hours, it may be helpful for the patient to remain relatively inactive and to sleep with the head elevated.

Movement

Movement of the graft over the wound bed before vascular attachment will tend to prevent these connections from forming. Movement of the graft in the period immediately after attachment may tear the small friable vessels, with resultant loss of a portion or all of the graft. The suture technique employed and choice of dressings are important in the prevention of movement-related complications. Most grafts can be made secure, so ambulation is permitted. Only occasionally will bed rest or hospitalization be required.

Exposed Bone and Cartilage

Occasionally, we are confronted with the problem of grafting a defect whose base contains denuded bone or cartilage. As these structures have no significant surface blood supply, large areas of exposed surface will not support a graft. A graft placed over small avascular defects, approximately one cm^2 or less, may survive via a bridging phenomenon, whereby nutritional support comes from the graft vessels overlying the adjacent vascularized bed until attachment is complete.

If there is exposed bone or cartilage sufficient to compromise a graft, there are several options that will aid in survival of the graft. Ideally, in this situation, it would be best to bring in a vascularized flap. However, assuming that a graft is used, exposed bone can be burred to expose vessels from the underlying spongy portion of the bone. On the ear, small holes can be cut through the exposed cartilage with a small 2.0 to 2.5 mm trephine to expose the vascularized perichondrium from the other side. At this point, the wound can often be grafted. Grafting can also be delayed until sufficient granulation tissue grows across the avascular tissue to support a graft. In this situation, the risk of infection is somewhat increased, and perioperative antibiotics may decrease the risk of wound infection.

Long-Term Complications

Long-term complications fall into two categories: functional and cosmetic.

Functional Complications

Functional complications relate primarily to the effects of wound contraction and graft fragility.

Even full thickness grafts can be expected to contract somewhat. The contraction probably occurs in the bed below the graft or in the layer of scar tissue sandwiched between the graft and the bed (Figs. 3-11 and 3-12). When grafting the eyelids, a graft 150 to 200 percent of the defect size is recommended, to overcompensate, in order to prevent ectropion formation.

In the event of wound contraction resulting in functional abnormality, a secondary revisional surgery may be necessary. This problem on the eyelid is usually treated by incising the graft at one edge, followed by wide undermining to release all of the tension, and then regrafting with a full thickness graft of 200 percent of the resulting defect.

Cosmetic Complications

Cosmetic problems after grafting usually relate to poor color and texture match or contour deformity.

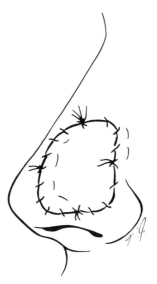

Figure 3-11

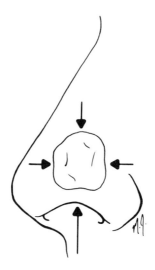

Figure 3-12

Since full thickness grafts will retain most of the qualities of the donor site, color and texture problems are minimal compared with split thickness grafts. Careful choices regarding these qualities at the time of surgery will prevent most of these problems. The most difficult sites to match are the nasal tip and the cutaneous upper lip. The reason for this involves the particular textural qualities of the skin in these locations, which are not easily found elsewhere.

Contour deformities can be a problem when grafting with a full thickness graft as compared with a split thickness graft. Minor differences between the thickness of graft and depth of defect will often even out with time. Significant differences between graft thickness and the depth of the defect may result in permanent deformity. An option for treatment of a deep defect is to delay grafting for a time (often 7 to 10 days), permitting granulation tissue to fill in the depth of the defect so a better contour can be achieved. In this situation, re-epithelialization will have usually begun. At the time of the delayed grafting, it is important to remove the new epidermis, returning the defect to its original boundaries before grafting.

The trapdoor or pincushion effect after surgery is related to wound contraction. This effect is caused by a layer of fibrosis that is laid down between the graft and the bed during the healing process. As this tissue contracts centrally, the graft is also pulled centrally. If the bed of the defect contracts more than the graft, the redundancy of the graft will be lifted upward, creating a bulging or pincushioning effect. The expectation of this problem is unpredictable but may be minimized with undermining beyond the boundaries of the defect. The problem may be persistent but, as the scar softens with time, the graft will flatten. The smoothing out of the graft may require months to a year or more. Intralesional steroids, injected into the fibrous layer below the graft, may speed the process via their collagenolytic activity. Only occasionally will a secondary surgical procedure be necessary to debulk the graft. Should this be necessary, an incision is made along one edge of the graft. Through the incision, the fibrous wafer of scar is removed. The deformity does not usually recur after such revisional surgery.

For slight elevation differences between graft and the surrounding skin, or for slightly depressed suture lines, focal dermabrasion can be an important, adjunctive modality. Dermabrasion is particularly effective on the nose, where depressed suture lines are common. Dermabrasion for scar revision can be performed under cryanesthesia, only, in most cases, without the addition of local anesthesia. A diamond fraise or wire brush is equally effective.

4

Composite Grafting

Unlike split thickness and full thickness skin grafts, which contain only skin, composite grafts contain two or more tissue layers. Examples of composite grafts include skin–fat, skin–cartilage, and skin–cartilage–skin grafts. The most common indications for composite grafts in dermatologic surgery are nasal alar and eyebrow reconstruction. These two techniques, specialized examples of skin grafting, are discussed in this chapter.

AURICULAR COMPOSITE GRAFTS FOR NASAL RECONSTRUCTION

Defects that involve the nasal alar rim are particularly difficult to reconstruct. There is insufficient adjacent skin on the nose for the development of local flaps. A variety of more distant flaps, using the nasolabial fold and forehead, have been described for alar reconstruction, but only rarely can they recreate the delicate thinness of the alar rim. Nasolabial flaps, often used for this purpose, frequently result in distortion of other features of the nose, such as the cheek–nose junction and, particularly, the alar groove, which must be crossed in moving such flaps to the ala.

Because of these limitations, grafts must frequently be considered for repair of alar rim defects. The auricular composite graft is particularly valuable for alar reconstruction. The auricular helix has a delicate curve similar to that of the alar rim, which permits its recreation. In addition, the cartilage that can be included in a composite graft taken from the ear serves to replace lost nasal cartilage or, at the very least, to provide structure to the graft, thereby decreasing wound contraction and the accompanying alar retraction.

Wound Healing Considerations

Unlike split and full thickness grafts, which obtain their nutrients and future blood supply from the base of the recipient bed, skin–cartilage–skin composite grafts are attached to the recipient site only at the graft edges. This means there is much less raw surface area available for revascularization between the composite graft and the recipient site. This necessarily limits the size of defect that can be repaired using a composite graft. The uppermost limit for such a graft has been recommended by various authors to be from 1 to 2 cm, such that no portion of the graft is further than 5 to 10 mm from any vascularized tissue. In general, composite grafting in other parts of the body is discouraged because of the vasculature required for supporting several tissue layers. Composite grafts for alar reconstruction is possible, however, because of the rich vascular supply that characterizes both the nose and the ear.

To increase the viability of grafts, it has been recommended that harvested grafts be placed in ice-chilled saline intraoperatively, with ice packs applied for several days postoperatively. The chilling, in theory, decreases the metabolic needs of the graft until revascularization has occurred and may increase viability.

Composite grafts routinely go through various stages during the healing process; patients must be informed of them so they will not be concerned about the appearance of the graft. McLaughlin is credited with documenting the changes that are routinely seen. Upon placement of the graft, the tissue appears dead white. At approximately 6 hours, the graft is noted to be a uniform, pale pink color, signifying that existing vessels from the graft have anastomosed with the surrounding recipient site vessels. At 12 to 24 hours, the graft appears deeply cyanotic, reflecting venous congestion, and at 3 to 7 days, the graft becomes a healthy pink color, denoting complete survival of the graft. Because of the tenuous nature of the vascular supply, all aspects of tissue handling, including meticulous but conservative, pinpoint hemostasis and careful suturing technique are all of critical importance for graft survival.

Donor Site Considerations

There are several donor sites available on the ear for harvesting composite grafts. It is important to appreciate the difference between them. The most common donor sites include the crus of the helix, the midhelical rim, and the lobe (Fig. 4-1). Recall that the auricular cartilage does not extend into the lobe; therefore a composite graft taken from the lobe will include only skin and fat. Grafts taken from the remainder of the ear can include cartilage as well, such that they represent a sandwich of skin–cartilage–skin.

There are several advantages to grafts harvested from the helical crus. The crus is straight, unlike the helical rim. In addition, the crus does not have an anterior roll, although this feature characterizes the helical rim. These factors make the helical crus my favorite donor site for alar reconstruction. The inner aspect of the crus, however, is shallow and, therefore, there is usually, at most, only a centimeter of trilaminar tissue (skin–cartilage–skin) available from this location. For alar defects of greater height, grafts taken from the

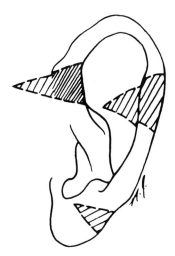

Figure 4-1

crus will not provide sufficient inner lining, and the helical rim will then need to be used as the donor, or other means of recreating the nasal inner lining will be needed.

The donor defect involving the crus can usually be repaired with minimal scar formation. A wedge excision from the helical rim tends to be more obvious, since the size of the ear will decrease.

Recipient Site Considerations

For longstanding, scarred-down, retracted alae, the tissue adjacent to the alar defect should be carefully debrided of scar tissue in order to assure the best possible blood supply for the composite graft. A tongue-in-groove inter-digitation of the graft edge into recipient site has been suggested to increase the amount of raw surface area exposed between the two tissues. For large defects, a turndown, hinged flap may be developed from the skin adjacent to the defect or from the nasal septum. This not only provides an inner lining to the nose but also further increases the surface area of the vascular bed.

Hemostasis is, of course, important, but should be handled conservatively. Large vessels should not be tied-off, but rather should be handled with precise, pinpoint electrocautery. Remaining small bleeders should be controlled with pressure only. Any char created from vigorous electrocoagulation, or any other foreign body present in the wound may have significant impact on revascularization.

TECHNIQUE

Local anesthesia is sufficient for both donor and recipient sites. Meticulous sterile surgical technique is mandatory.

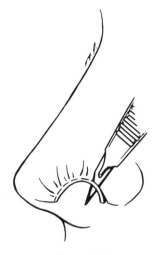

Figure 4-2

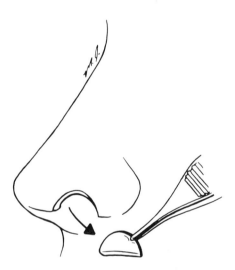

Figure 4-3

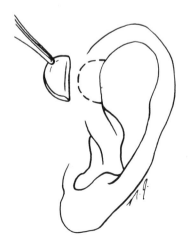

Figure 4-4

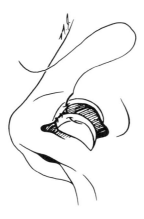

Figure 4-5

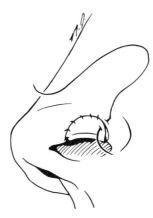

Figure 4-6

Step 1. If the alar defect is longstanding, it must be adequately prepared for grafting. The scarred-down rim is carefully excised to expose a vascular rich, raw surface for grafting (Fig. 4-2).

Step 2. The defect is carefully measured and a template is made to the exact size of the defect (Fig. 4-3). This prevents miscalculations. The proposed graft is marked on the donor site (Fig. 4-4).

Step 3. The graft is carefully harvested. When it is necessary to grasp the tissue, a skin hook is used, rather than pick-ups, as this will minimize tissue injury. The graft is then placed on ice-cold, sterile, saline-soaked gauze until ready for placement.

Step 4. The graft is then carefully sutured in two layers. The undersurface of the graft, which will replace the inner lining of the nose, is secured first. A 6-0 absorbable suture is used (Fig. 4-5).

Step 5. The skin is then closed with 6-0 nonabsorbable sutures. It is not necessary to suture the cartilage. Since there should be no tension across the lines of closure, very small bites should be taken through the tissue with each stitch (Fig. 4-6). This will help minimize vessel strangulation and thereby maximize potential available vessels for re-anastomosis.

A Vaseline gauze dressing is placed in the nasal vestibule for internal support, and a light coating of antibiotic ointment is placed on the external suture line. No external dressing is necessary, although a Telfa or thin gauze dressing is recommended in order to provide protection from external injury.

Ice packs should be applied to the grafted site as frequently as possible during the immediate postoperative period and up to several days afterward. Antibiotics are not always indicated but, considering the normal inherent colonization of the area by bacteria, oral antibiotics are almost always given. Sutures are removed at 1 week.

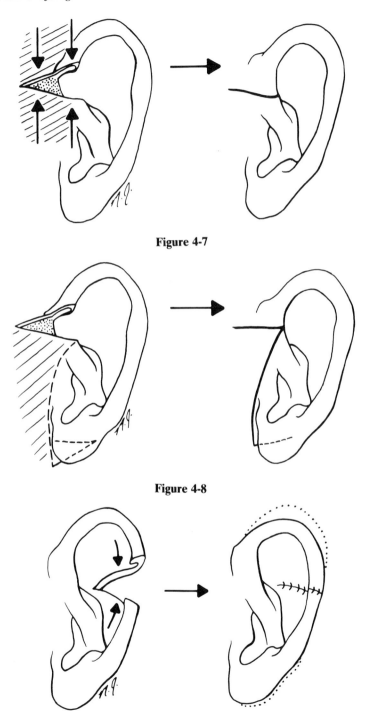

Figure 4-7

Figure 4-8

Figure 4-9

Closure of the Donor Site

Helical crus defects may be repaired in one of several ways. The local tissues may be simply undermined, and the defect closed in a side-to-side manner by advancing the tissues from above and below (Fig. 4-7). Because of the underlying cartilage, primary closure may not be possible. A flap or graft repair may become necessary.

A Burow's triangle advancement flap, based inferiorly and medially is most useful (Fig. 4-8). An inferiorly based advancement flap, or rotation flap based inferiorly and posteriorly, will also close this defect. A full thickness graft may also be indicated and can be taken from the postauricular sulcus. Helical rim and lobe defects are closed in the same manner as any wedge resection of the ear (Fig. 4-9).

HAIR-BEARING STRIP GRAFTS FOR EYEBROW RECONSTRUCTION

The eyebrows represent an important aesthetic and functional anatomic feature of the central face. A loss of one or both brows creates a significant cosmetic deformity. Because of this, patients are often quite eager to undergo reconstruction.

The most common causes of cicatricial alopecia of the eyebrows includes thermal burns and other injuries to the face, surgical removal in the treatment of benign or malignant tumors, and radiation exposure. Reconstruction is usually possible after all forms of traumatic loss.

A variety of techniques has been described for reconstruction of the eyebrow. These include punch grafting, single hair transplantation, hair-bearing pedicle flaps, and strip grafting. Strip grafting is probably the most commonly used method, since it can be performed under local anesthesia, usually requires only a single procedure, and the results are usually quite satisfactory.

Strip grafts used for eyebrow reconstruction are generally taken from the scalp. Since the hair follicles are located in the subcutaneous tissue below the dermis, a graft that is intended to include growing hair must contain both skin and fat. Therefore, strip grafts represent a type of composite graft.

Recipient Site Considerations

Examination of the normal eyebrow reveals that the pattern of hair growth is multidirectional. At the most medial portion of the brow, the hair grows in an upward and sometimes medial direction. The hair in the lateral two-thirds of the brow is angled laterally. In addition, there are some inferiorly oriented hairs at the most posterolateral portion of the brow (Fig. 4-10).

In men, the eyebrow normally overlies the orbital rim. In women, the normal location of the brow is slightly above the orbital rim. Many factors influence the precise location of the brow and the aging process results in

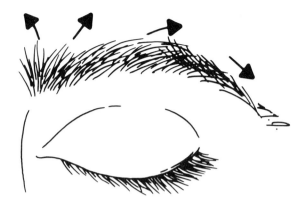

Figure 4-10

brow ptosis in most individuals. When attempting to recreate both brows, these issues must be considered. When replacing only a single brow, the shape and height of the contralateral brow serves as the model. The eyebrow in men is often thicker than in women. Therefore, the density and coarseness of the hair must also be evaluated.

The ultimate survival of the graft may depend on the quality of the blood supply in the recipient site. This is particularly important when the cause of alopecia is traumatic. Severe scarring, with its associated diminished blood supply, may limit the size of graft that can be placed. For a severely scarred recipient site, some authors have suggested that the graft be limited to 5 mm in height. Otherwise, a graft of 1 cm in height may survive, if there is minimal to no scarring present at the recipient site.

Donor Site Considerations

The scalp, with its nearly unlimited supply of donor tissue, serves as the donor site for strip grafting for eyebrow reconstruction. Scalp hair density and coarseness generally increases from the temple posteriorly to the occipital scalp. The choice of the appropriate donor site depends on the hair quality desired. The transplanted hair will grow at the same rate as does the scalp hair. Trimming of the brow hair will therefore be required every 2 to 3 weeks.

At the donor site, the proposed graft is planned such that the long axis of the graft is in a cephalocaudal direction, with the medial portion of the graft most cephalad (Fig. 4-11). After transfer, this places the orientation of the hair growth in a uniformly lateral direction. While this does not recreate the multidirectional growth pattern of the natural eyebrow, it creates a fairly normal appearance, since the predominant direction of growth of the natural brow is lateral.

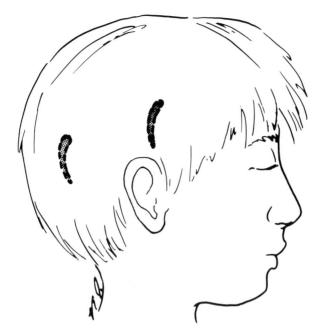

Figure 4-11

TECHNIQUE

Strip grafting can be performed in the office under local anesthesia. The usual plastic surgical instrumentation is used.

Step 1. The proposed brow is planned and marked on the patient. A template of the exact shape of the proposed brow is made.

Step 2. The donor site is chosen based on density and coarseness of the hair desired. The hair at the donor site is trimmed so that the remaining hair is several millimeters in length. The donor site should not be shaved, as the orientation of the remaining hair permits accurate angling of the incision, so that it is parallel to the hair shafts and underlying hair bulbs. Using the template, the dimensions of the proposed graft is marked on the donor site.

Step 3. The donor site is prepped and infiltrated with the local anesthetic agent. As mentioned, it is critical that the incision be made parallel to the hair shafts, to prevent injury to the underlying hair follicles (Fig. 4-12). The incision is carried through the fat and galea to the periosteum. The graft is then placed in a Petri dish containing sterile, saline-soaked gauze. *Note:* A small layer of subcutaneous fat is necessary to cover the deeper aspects of the follicles, in order to ensure survival of the hair. It is easier to trim the graft of galea and

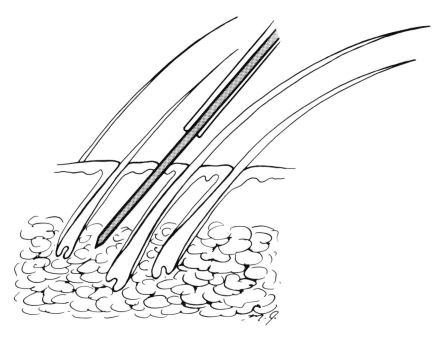

Figure 4-12

excess fat after removal from the donor site rather than during the removal, when the normal bleeding tends to obscure the appropriate plane of dissection.

Step 4. The donor site can then be converted into a fusiform shape as needed, and closed. A layered closure is used. The galea is secured with 2-0 or 3-0 absorbable sutures and the skin may be closed with 3-0 nylon sutures. I prefer a running locked stitch.

Step 5. The recipient site is then prepped, draped, and infiltrated with local anesthetic. Skin is removed to create the appropriately shaped recipient site for the strip graft. Meticulous hemostasis is important, and it is critically important to handle the tissue delicately, in order to preserve all available vascularity. Next, the graft is placed into the defect and closed with 6-0 nylon sutures. An interrupted or running stitch may be used, as desired (Fig. 4-13). A topical antibiotic ointment and light pressure dressing are indicated. Sutures may be removed in 1 week.

In case of a partial loss of the graft, a second strip graft may be placed. If the loss is only spotty, small punch grafts may be used. When there is a question, it is better to place the graft slightly too low rather than too high on the brow. It is simpler to excise a strip of skin above the graft and elevate its location than it is to lower it.

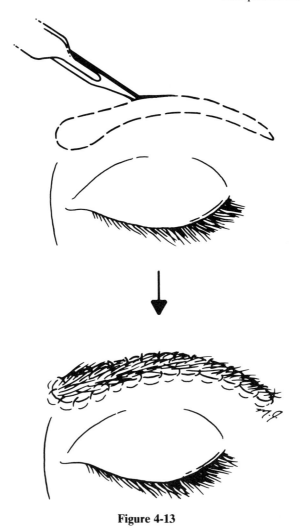

Figure 4-13

In summary, strip grafting for eyebrow reconstruction represents a practical and relatively simple modification of full thickness grafting techniques for eyebrow reconstruction. The results can be gratifying in patients who have suffered loss of one or both eyebrows.

Index

Page numbers followed by f indicate figures; those followed by t indicate tables.